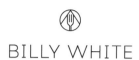

BILLY WHITE

EAT RUN ENJOY

photography PATRIK ENGSTRÖM

BLOOMSBURY SPORT

LONDON · OXFORD · NEW YORK · NEW DELHI · SYDNEY

BLOOMSBURY SPORT
Bloomsbury Publishing Plc
50 Bedford Square, London, WC1B 3DP, UK

BLOOMSBURY, BLOOMSBURY SPORT and the Diana logo are trademarks of
Bloomsbury Publishing Plc

First published in 2019 in Sweden as *Eat, Run, Enjoy* by Gawell Förlag
First published in Great Britain 2021

A catalogue record for this book is available from the British Library

Library of Congress Cataloguing-in-Publication data has been applied for
add where a UK originated single-ISBN edition for which we own US rights

ISBN: HB: 978-1-4729-8606-1; eBook: 978-1-4729-8607-8

2 4 6 8 10 9 7 5 3 1

Printed and bound in China by C&C Offset Printing Co., Ltd

Bloomsbury Publishing Plc makes every effort to ensure that the papers used in the
manufacture of our books are natural, recyclable products made from wood grown in well-
managed forests. Our manufacturing processes conform to the environmental regulations of
the country of origin.

To find out more about our authors and books visit www.bloomsbury.com
and sign up for our newsletters

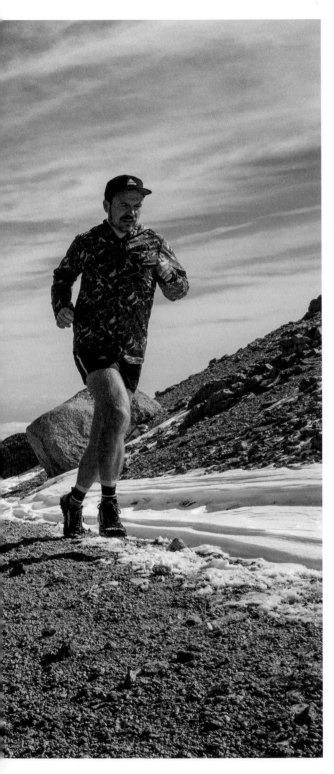

Contents

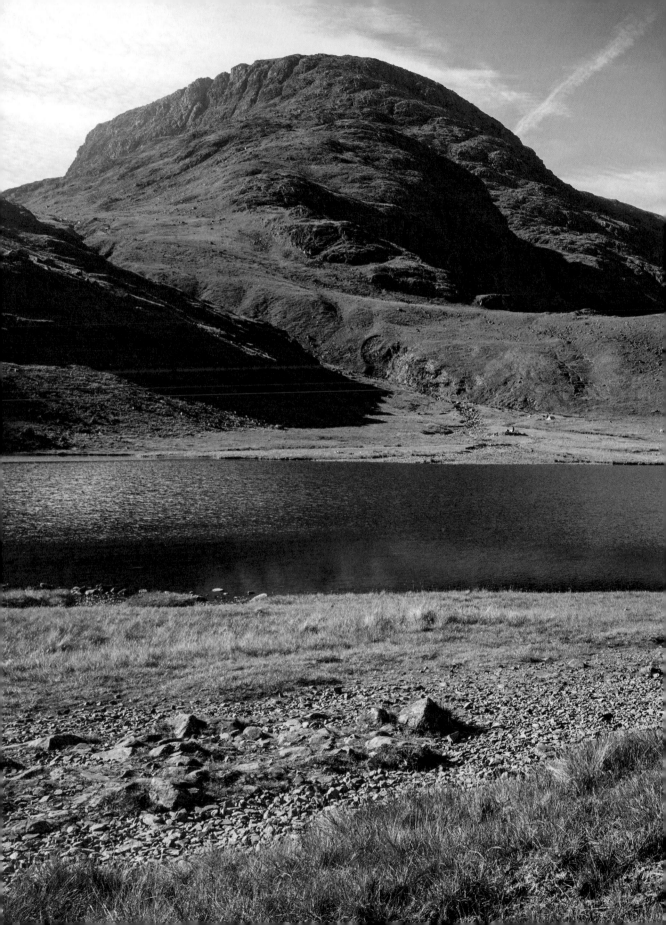

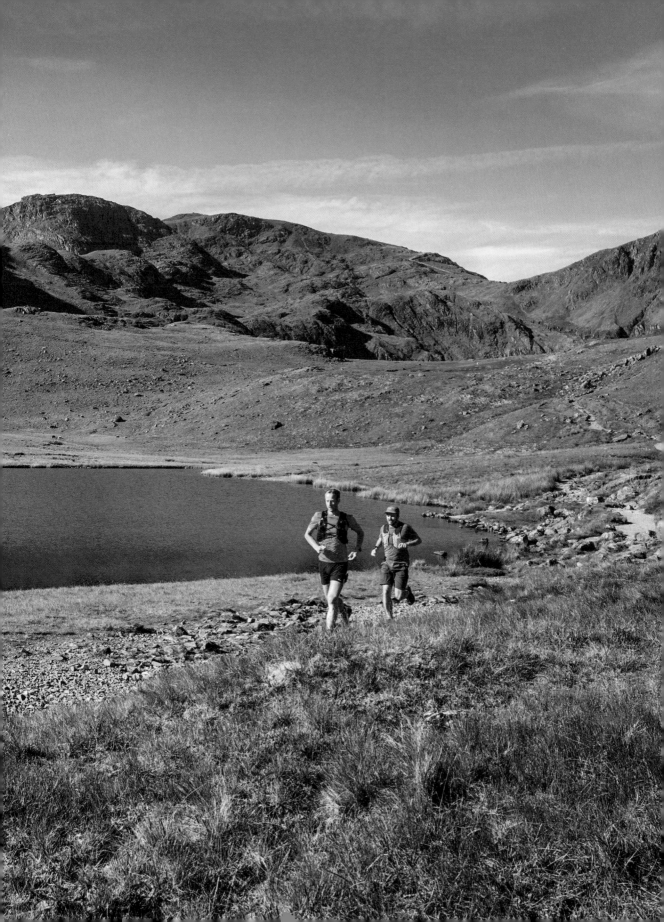

Introduction

This book is about my two passions: trail running and delicious food. There are hundreds of books on the market about training for running or how to eat for peak performance, but not so many that focus on the enjoyment of food and how that can coincide with the enjoyment of running, or any exercise for that matter. I wanted to bring together some of my favourite recipes – all easy-to-make and nutritionally balanced – that I believe will help runners of all levels of ability to reach their performance goals in a delicious and enjoyable way.

Over the last few years, I've also been fortunate enough to be able to spend time with some of the best trail and mountain runners in the world, hearing their nutritional advice and tips on how to become a better runner. So, dotted throughout the book are stories about some of my encounters with them, sharing what I learned.

As a runner, a father and a chef, I want to eat in the best way possible, so that I can fully appreciate life. I hope this book will inspire you, both with ideas to cook up tasty and healthy food in the kitchen, as well as to get outside and enjoy some time on the trails.

My Story

I started running just over seven years ago. I was creeping up to thirty and years of long days in the kitchen, combined with a bad diet and lots of afterwork beers, had started to catch up with me. It wasn't an overnight thing, but I realised something had to give.

After leading a very active lifestyle as a young man – skateboarding, snowboarding and even kickboxing – as soon as I found my passion for cooking, all these things took a back seat, eventually disappearing from my life by my early twenties. For me, food was a revelation, life changing! For many years, all I cared about was food: cooking and eating; focusing on every detail I could about life in the kitchen; working long days and winding down with long nights in the bar; learning what I could from each chef I worked for and moving on to the next. I've been very lucky to work at some of the most well-respected restaurants in the world and worked side by side with some of the industry's best chefs.

Then, in 2011, with a bit of prompting from a close friend, I signed up for a half marathon, and from that moment on I continued to run. I loved everything about it, from the feeling it gave me, to the fact that, as a father of two small kids, working in a demanding industry, it suited my schedule – finding the time to go to the gym or play football would be a real struggle for me. In many ways, endurance running and high-end cooking are similar: they take a lot of training; you spend many hours of the day on your feet; there is no guarantee

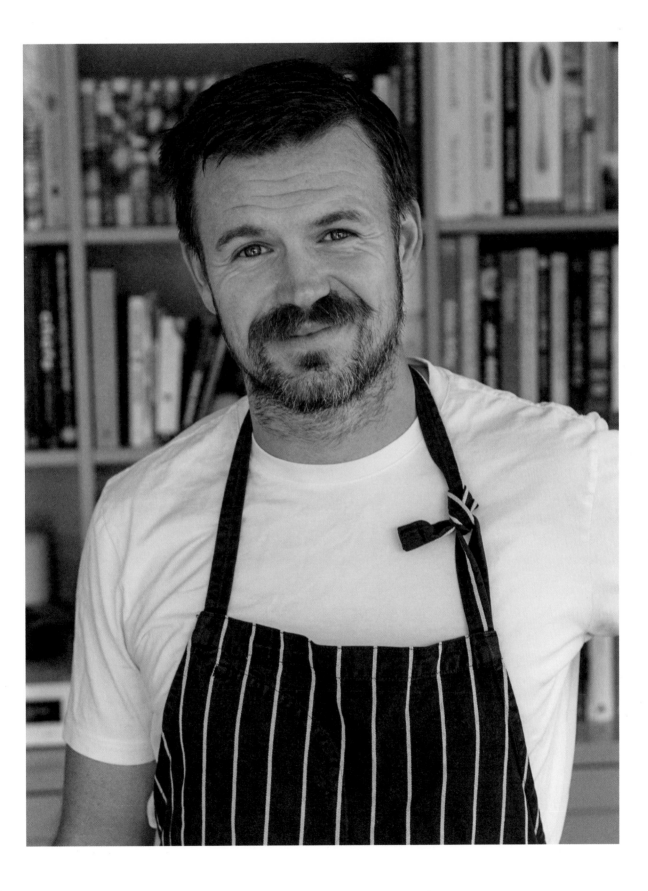

of success; but the journey is as important as the goal.

From a practical point of view, standing for many years for many hours in the kitchen actually gave me a good base for spending long days out on the trail – it's not a training method I would recommend, but you get the idea!

From the first day, the hills and countryside trails were always my preferred place to run – that connection to nature and the freedom you feel when you're away from it all is something that makes the daily grind all the more manageable.

And then, of course, I came back to considering food. Since starting to run, there is no doubt that the way I cook has evolved. In the fine dining restaurants of the late 1990s, where I learned to cook, the food was always quite heavy. Over the years, trends have changed, meals have become lighter and vegetables so much more appreciated, which has opened up a style of cooking that is much more beneficial to the health of the eater.

Nowadays, I find myself looking more to Southern Europe, North Africa and the Middle East for inspiration. A lot of the basic ingredients are familiar, but it's their use of fresh herbs and spices that gives everything such a welcome lift. I've brought many of these recipes to the book as they are so delicious and different while still offering all the nutritional benefits a runner needs. Turkish Scrambled Eggs (p.33), Polenta with Peas, Pecorino and Almonds (p.131), Spiced Lamb with Roast Aubergine (p.119) and Roast Chicken with Quinoa Tabbouleh and Chicory (p.116) are some great examples, and there are many more.

Meeting the Ultra Runners

When I decided to write this book, I felt I had no choice but to try to get some elite runners involved. Trail running is not your average sport; with races ranging from a couple of miles straight up boggy fells in the Lake District to over 200 miles (320km) circumnavigating Lake Tahoe in the US and absolutely everything in between. I've cooked for my whole career, and while nutrition is important to me, when it comes to the specifics of how it works for sport, I could – at best – call myself a keen amateur. The only way of getting a balanced overview of dietary and lifestyle advice was to try to get the opinions from a broad spectrum of runner.

I couldn't be happier with the runners who agreed to be involved in this book. Emelie Forsberg (Sweden), Ida Nilsson (Sweden), Mimmi Kotka (Sweden), Ricky Lightfoot (UK), Courtney Dauwalter (USA) and Zach Miller (USA) all agreed to let me come and run with them and it was fascinating to get an insight into how they train and eat, and – most importantly – to see just how much they enjoy trail running.

Interestingly, all the athletes displayed varying degrees of interest in food; from Emelie, Ida and Mimmi, who are so into food they've set up their own nutrition brand and talk about very little else; to Courtney Dauwalter, who – whilst enjoying eating and watching that she doesn't eat too much junk – actually has very little interest in cooking and loves tacos, candy and beer (!); and if you follow Zach Miller on social media, you'll know that he has a lot of fun eating and sometimes takes his mantra 'eating is training' to whole new levels (there was certainly no leftover apple pie at Barr Camp when he had finished!). However, the energy all the athletes put into understanding that good food is an essential part of their training is the same.

Ultra runners often adhere to very specific diets and stay on strict training schedules, but I noticed that among the runners I met this really wasn't the case. They were all very in tune with their bodies, of course, and they trained hard and ran a lot, but not without carefully listening to any warning signs from their bodies and paying close attention to any niggle; taking it easy when necessary and only pushing when things feel good.

Another key lesson they taught me was the importance of patience. Running ultra marathons is enormously demanding on the body, and building up to these distances doesn't happen overnight. Courtney Dauwalter ran her first 50K (31-mile) race in 2011. After failure at her first 100-mile (160km) race in 2012, she persevered and eventually completed that distance one year later. She has spent the six years since pushing the boundaries of what's possible, with very little injury. It is testament to how a careful and steady approach works.

Eating for Running

All my experience as a chef and a runner has taught me that just as taste is a very individual thing, so is what your body needs. There are no set rules to fuelling for endurance running races or for all the heavy training you need to do beforehand; instead – and maybe this is the most fun part – you need to experiment and continually try new things whilst training, or in the lead-up to a race, to find what works for you.

After seven years of running, I'm finally beginning to understand what works for me and what really doesn't. For instance, I know that I struggle with rice; if I eat any more than just a very small portion, I feel bloated for a long time afterwards, so I'll always avoid it if I know I'm going to train later that day. Try out the recipes in this book and see how you feel – adjusting portion sizes to suit your appetite and needs. I've suggested which recipes I think work well for certain points in your day, whether you are training, racing or recovering, and there are a few ideas in the menu planners on pp.14–15.

I know I said there are no set rules but actually there is one: eating something immediately after a training session is a must. This is not an excuse to completely stuff your face, but you do need to give the body a quick fix when energy is at a low. There are plenty of tips in this book for suitable snacks and quick meals for any time of the day.

Later on in the afternoon or evening after training, when you may not want a big meal, the Banana, Almond Butter and Chia Smoothie (p.199) or Greek Yogurt with Apple, Honey, Olive Oil and Salt (p.163) are quick and easy ways to give you some much-needed energy, rather than having a heavy meal sitting in your stomach late in the day.

Enjoying the Run

I'm sure Ricky Lightfoot isn't at his happiest whilst running his weekly road intervals or doing a speed session on the treadmill, but it helps him to do what he loves most of all: moving quickly over the the fells of the Lake District. All the runners I met were competitive – of course, you don't reach the level they have if you're not – but that alone isn't what spurs them on. It's the thoughts of mountain trails that gets them up at 5 a.m. on a rainy November morning. That sense of dedication to the joy of the run came through stronger than any relationship to food or training or winning races.

I ran my first trail race in 2013 and since then I've completed my first 100-mile (160km) race. It has been a long journey. I've raced everything from road-based 10Ks to 100K in the jungles of Thailand, to 130K deep in the Swedish forest during the winter. I've met many wonderful people and I know that, as long as I continue to run, I'll meet many many more. The overriding thing I learned on this journey was not just to be mindful of what you eat, but – more importantly – to **do what you love**.

This is really what the 'Enjoy' part of my book title represents – you've got to love it to do it: enjoy the running and enjoy eating delicious real food. Just as you shouldn't push yourself too far with the training, don't punish yourself by forcing down 'athlete's' protein powders or foods you don't really like. Conversely, don't undo all your hard work with excessive amounts of junk food or empty calories either. Whether you like to run an occasional 5K in your local woods or multi-day ultra races, the advice is pretty much the same: if you listen to your body, and if are enjoying yourself, you can't really go wrong.

Billy White

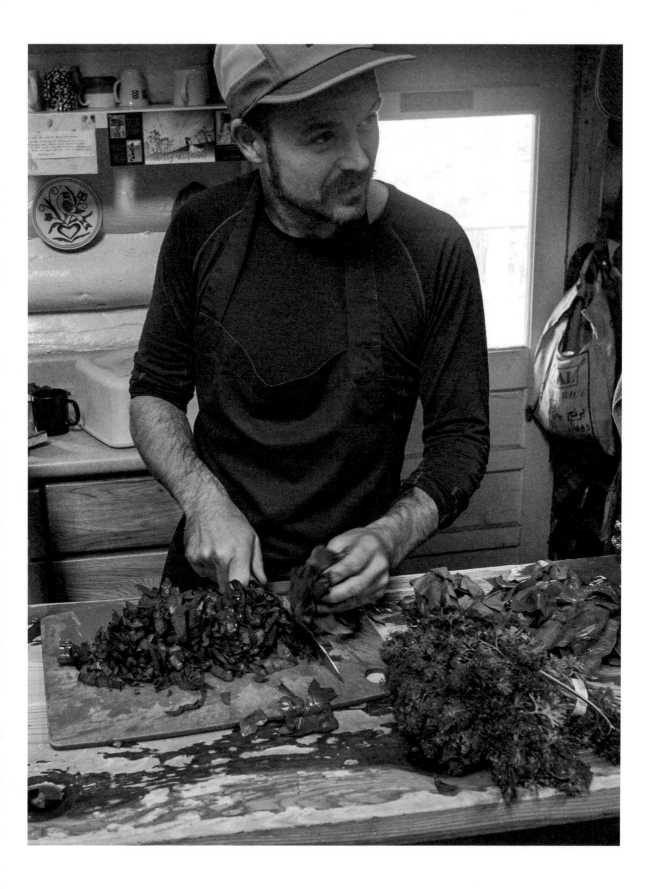

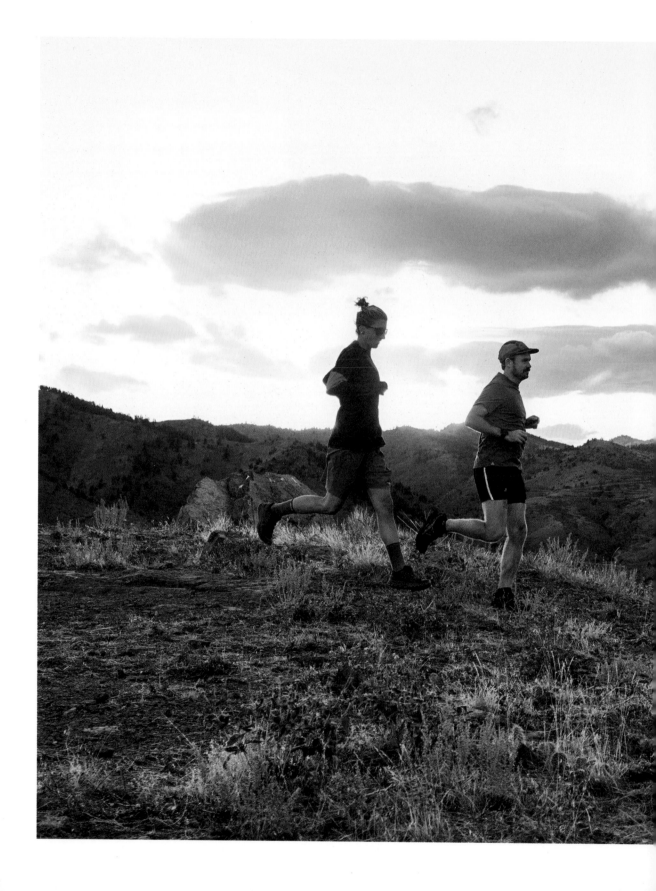

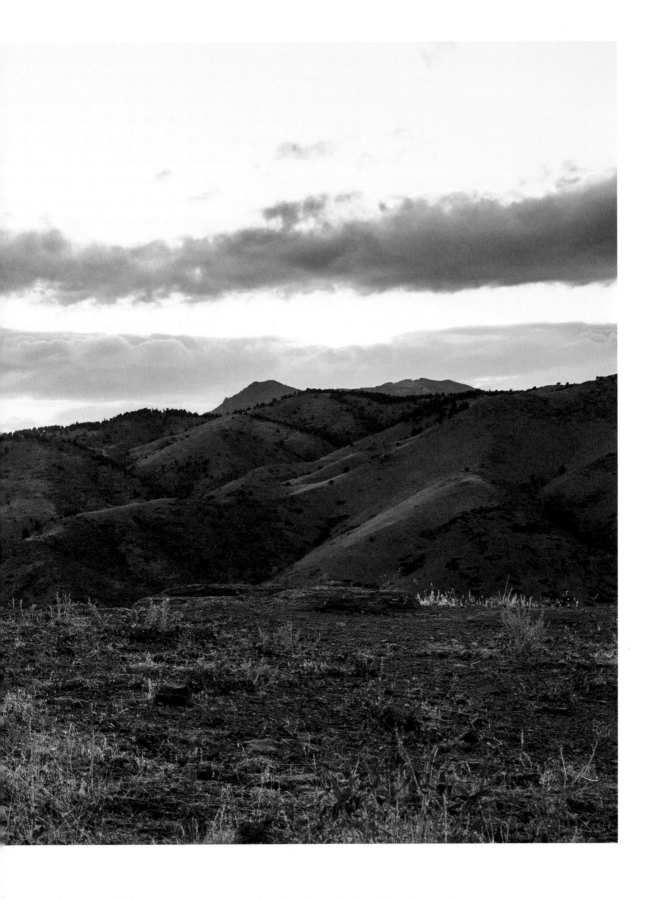

Menu Planner

Planning a menu for the week can be a bit tricky. Generally, I like to eat most of my carbs earlier in the day and finish with something a bit lighter. Most of the meals in this book will work for big training days as well as rest days; it depends a lot on how you are feeling. Here are a few examples of daily meal plans that have worked for me.

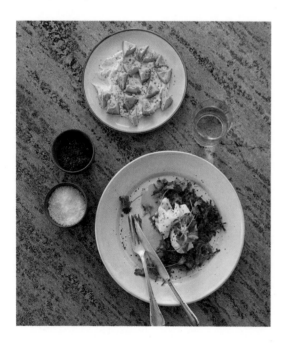

Pre-race day/Training day

BREAKFAST: Rye and Oat Porridge with Blueberry Chia Compote (p.23).

LUNCH: Choose something quite light, but with a good amount of slow-burning carbohydrates. Try: Rainbow Trout, Potato and Egg Salad (p.89) or Tuscan Bean Soup (p.74).

AFTERNOON SNACK: Chilli and Thyme Seed Bars (p.214).

DINNER: The traditional pre-race meal of a giant bowl of pasta is always too much for me; a few times I've stood on the start line and felt bloated from the previous evening's meal. Try choosing dishes that are high in carbs but balanced with a lot of other vegetables so you don't get overly full, such as Cod with Curried Coconut Leeks (p.124) or Roast Chicken with Quinoa Tabbouleh and Chicory (p.116). For dessert, a slice of Dark Chocolate and Beetroot Cake (p.160) is a good way to get in a few last-minute carbs the evening before a race.

Race day

BREAKFAST: Rye and Oat Porridge with Blueberry Chia Compote (p.23) or Nut Butter and Banana on Toast (p.200).

LUNCH: For late-starting races you might like a light lunch such as **Watermelon, Charred Asparagus and Feta Salad** (p.80) or the **Roast Cauliflower, Chickpea, Olive and Pomegranate Salad with Hummus** (p.84)

However, races are often in the middle of the day, so skip lunch and pack a few portions of the **Ecotrail Raw Slice** (p.216) or a **Raw Breakfast Slice** (p.217) in your pack. I also always have a **Chilli and Thyme Seed Bar** (p.214) and a bag of **Trail Mix** (p.218), in case I crave something not-so-sweet.

DINNER: After a race is when I allow myself anything I want! It's very rare that I'll cook for myself after a race, but if I do it will be something like Flank **Steak with Fermented Red Slaw, Labneh and Sweet Potato Wedges** (p.122). More often than not, I just crave a burger and a few beers.

Post-race day/Recovery

BREAKFAST: Sweet Potato Rosti with Poached Eggs (p.29), Tahini Yogurt with Avocado and Sesame (p.30) or Steak and Eggs with Purple Sprouting Broccoli and Jalapeños (p.34) – all contain the carbs your body will be craving after a race effort, plus plenty of protein to help recovery, and iron, which is also necessary when the body is fatigued.

LUNCH: Try something soothing like **Chicken and Leek Broth** (p.67) with some freshly baked **Basic Sourdough Bread** (p.185).

DINNER: Choose a quick and easy recipe, so you don't have to spend too much time hobbling around the kitchen on achy legs. **Spaghetti with Cavolo Nero and Walnut Pesto** (p.134) is really simple. I find the last thing I want the day after a race is dessert, especially after all the sweet things you tend to eat during a race, but if you have a sweeter tooth than me, I'd recommend **Blueberry and Honey Frozen Yogurt with Mint and Fresh Blueberries** (p.156) – another simple recipe to reduce time on your feet.

(Very) Basic Diet Advice for Runners

Taking advice on what you should eat, how much of it and how often is a bit of a murky area, in my opinion. Things that work for some people absolutely don't work for others. There are so many diets out there: high-fat-low-carb-ketogenic; high-carb-low-fat; you can be advised to feed yourself small meals many times throughout the day; or fast for eighteen hours and stuff your face for the remaining six... It's a minefield! Similarly, the clean eating movement **should** be a good thing, but it's easily taken too far, especially if you place a lot of physical demands on yourself in training.

One thing I do know: you need to eat plenty when you run a lot.

I don't think that you can eat as much as you want of whatever you want, but you certainly need to eat a little extra. The portion sizes of the recipes in this book can easily be adjusted to suit your appetite and most dishes can be tweaked to your tastes, without compromising flavour.

It's important to stress that the recipes in this book are not intended to offer a complete runner's diet or to be used for specific weight loss, but they do constitute a healthy, balanced and natural diet if you plan on running regularly for pleasure or competition. If you are running to lose weight, I would recommend looking into tailored diets and training plans and taking advice from your doctor or another nutritional professional.

Initially, I started running without a great deal of diet change. I lost a few kilos but, over time, even though my running mileage was consistently quite high (around 50–80km/31–50 miles per week), I was always a little heavier than I would have liked. Only in the last year or so have I dropped the last 5–6kg (11–13lbs) that I wanted to lose. I occasionally run my morning commute on an empty stomach, but I think that introducing one to two dedicated speed or hill sessions every week and including two to three brief strength workouts, focusing on the core muscles, helped me shed those last few kilos.

I am also an advocator of eating natural whole foods. It was reading the small book *Food Rules* by Michael Pollan that had a big effect on the way I eat. His simple and often amusing tips, such as 'eat food, not too much, mostly plants' or 'don't eat anything your great grandmother wouldn't recognise as food' are priceless. One of my personal favourites is: 'eat foods made from ingredients that you can picture in their raw state or growing in nature.' It's great advice, whether you run or not. •

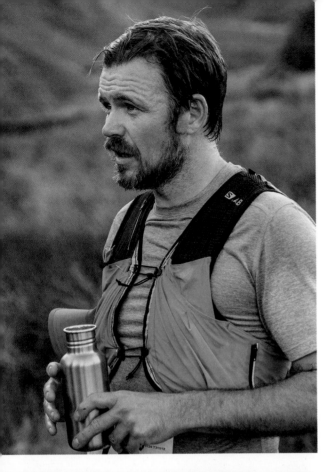

Tips

REFUEL. Always have something ready for when you have just finished a run, even if it's a just a glass of milk or a banana. Immediately after training is when you need to restore glycogen to reduce muscle breakdown.

STAY HYDRATED. Thirst is a very good indicator of whether you need a drink or not, but it's important to stay on top of hydration when running or exercising in general. If I'm planning on running for longer than 1 hour, I'll generally bring a water bottle with me.

DON'T BUY JUNK FOOD. If you don't have crisps and snacks at home, it's so much harder to eat them. Nuts and fruits are perfect substitutes. Also, never go shopping when you are hungry! It's a sure-fire way to end up with a shopping basket full of things that may not be the best for you. I try to plan the week's meals ahead and then do the grocery shop online with home delivery – this saves time and reduces temptation.

TRY TO KEEP A GOOD BALANCE. If you look at your meals over the course of a day, they should generally be made up of 50–60 per cent carbs, 15–20 per cent protein and 20–25 per cent fats. I probably go slightly lighter on the carbs a couple of days a week, but that's after a few years of getting to know what works best for me. Try to go for slow-release wholegrain carbs, such as oats or quinoa, or carb-rich vegetables such as sweet potato and beetroot (beets). Think about vegetable-based proteins, such as pulses; they can be a good alternative to meat. When it comes to fat, unsaturated fats such as extra-virgin olive oil and rapeseed oil are great, but don't be afraid of a little butter from time to time.

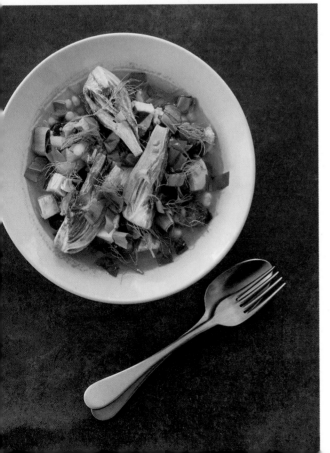

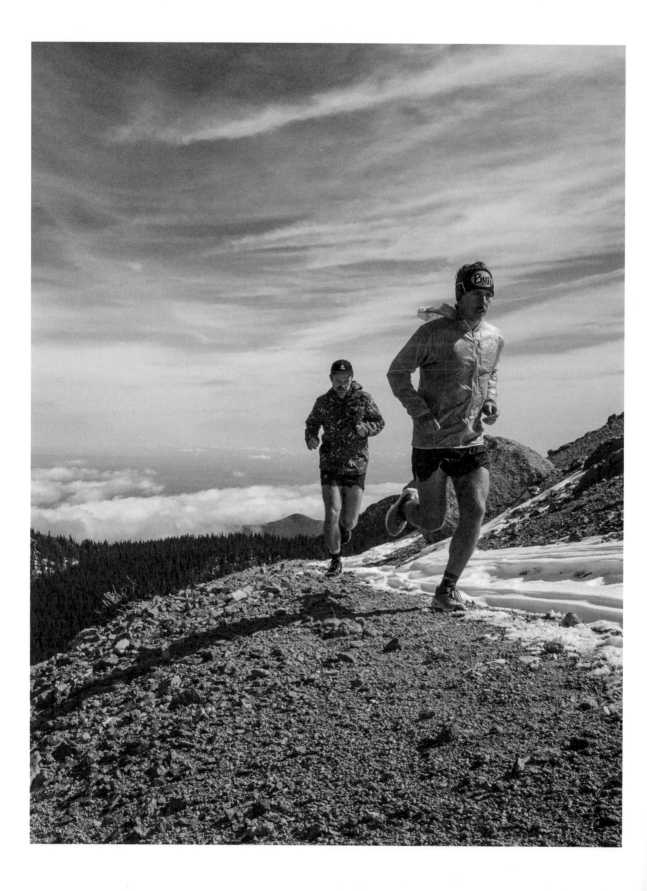

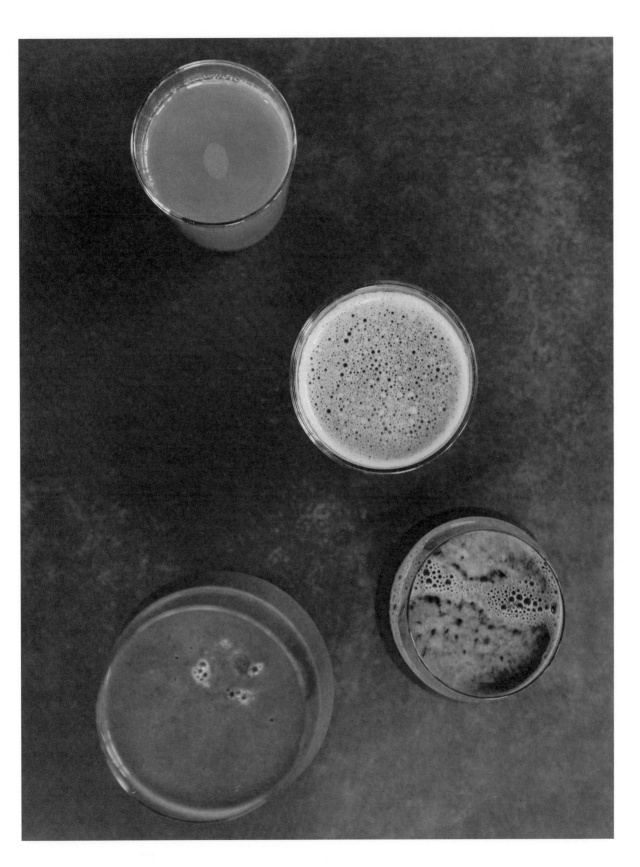

CHAPTER ONE

Breakfast

———

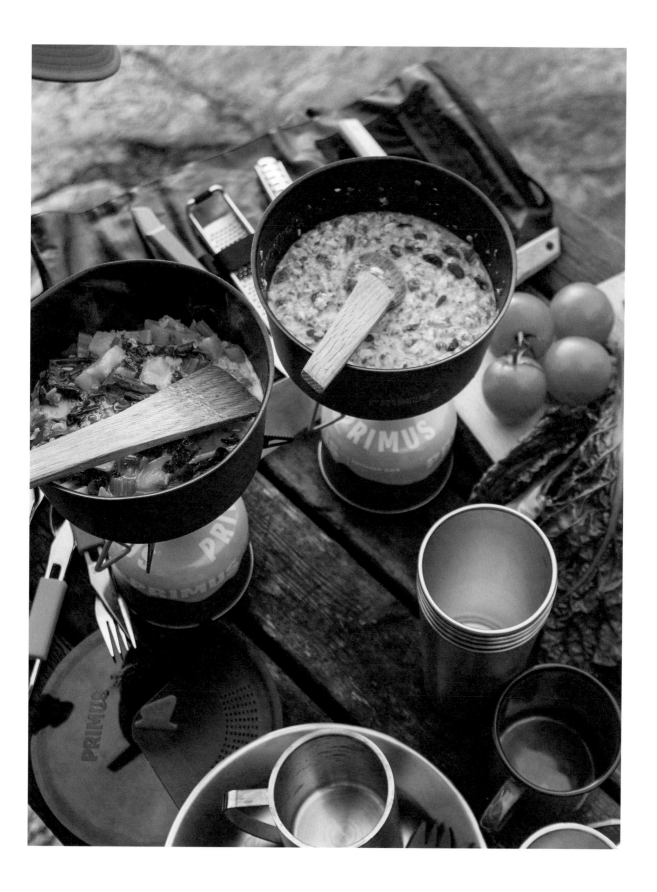

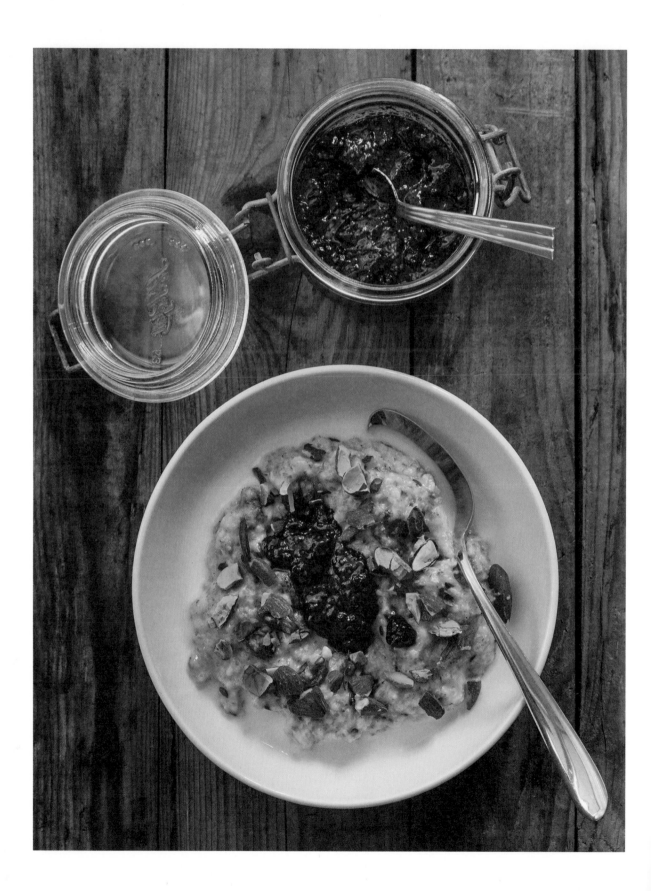

A great start to the day, I will generally have this on race-day mornings. I don't normally measure in cups, but this is the easiest way to make this. When you buy the oats and rye, empty the bags into a bowl and mix the two together – it saves messing about every morning.

RYE AND OAT PORRIDGE
(WALTER'S SUPER PORRIDGE)

SERVES 1

90g (3¼oz or ¾ cup) mixed rye and rolled oats
1 tbsp flax seeds
1 tsp chia seeds
2 tbsp raisins
a pinch of salt
475ml (2 cups) milk, plus extra to serve
250ml (1 cup) water
Blueberry Chia Compote (see right) and
    chopped toasted almonds, to serve

1. Combine all the ingredients in a saucepan over a medium heat and gently cook for about 5 minutes, stirring frequently to stop it catching, until the porridge is smooth and the oats and rye have broken down. If it looks as though it is drying out, add a little more milk.

2. Serve in a bowl with a little milk poured over, topped with a big spoonful of blueberry chia compote, and a scattering of chopped toasted almonds for some crunch.

This makes a large quantity, but it freezes really well, so I always make much more than I need and freeze it into small portions that will last a few days when defrosted.

BLUEBERRY CHIA COMPOTE

MAKES 1 LITRE (4 CUPS)

1kg (2¼lb) fresh blueberries
300g (11oz) golden caster sugar
100g (3¾oz) chia seeds

1. Place the blueberries in a saucepan and gently bring to a simmer. Cook for 2–3 minutes until the berries have released their juices, then add the sugar and simmer until the sugar has dissolved, around 5 minutes. Remove from the heat, stir in the chia seeds and allow to cool.

2. When cooled, pour into small airtight containers and freeze, or store in the refrigerator for up to 1 week.

Labneh is a soft cheese made from strained yogurt and it is really easy to make at home. I use it in many forms: with fresh fruits or nuts as a brunch dish; as a dip with za'atar and olive oil for a mezze-style starter; or as a side to spiced slowed-cooked lamb or a chickpea stew. It's really versatile and so delicious.

LABNEH WITH POMEGRANATE, WALNUTS AND MINT

SERVES 4

1 pomegranate
400g (14oz) Labneh (see right)
100g (3¾oz) toasted walnuts, chopped
a handful of fresh mint, coarsely chopped
a drizzle of good-quality fruity olive oil
sea salt flakes, to taste

1. Score the outer shell of the pomegranate and peel away the tough skin.

2. Gently pick out the seeds – it's laborious but it's worth it for a bowl of ruby-red jewels. Alternatively, submerge the scored pomegranate in a bowl of water and pull it apart, releasing the seeds with your hands. The pith will float and can be discarded; the seeds will sink and can be strained out.

3. Spread a good spoonful of labneh over the bottom of 4 serving bowls and scatter with the pomegranate seeds, chopped walnuts and mint. Drizzle over a little olive oil and finish with a pinch of salt, to taste.

LABNEH WITH CITRUS FRUIT

SERVES 4

1 blood orange
1 navel orange
1 pink grapefruit
400g (14oz) Labneh (see below)
a drizzle of good-quality fruity olive oil
sea salt flakes, to taste

1. Using a sharp knife, peel the skin from the fruit, removing as much of the white pith as possible. Cut into bite-size pieces and remove any pips.

2. Spread a good spoonful of labneh over the bottom of 4 serving bowls and arrange the citrus fruit on top. Serve, drizzled with a little olive oil and a pinch of salt, to taste.

LABNEH

MAKES 400G (14OZ)

500g (1¼lb) full-fat Greek yogurt
a pinch of salt

1. Mix the yogurt and salt in a bowl – it shouldn't be very salty, just lightly seasoned. Pour into a sieve lined with a double layer of muslin or a very fine cheesecloth and place it over a bowl. Place in the refrigerator for 4–6 hours until the yogurt in the cloth has become thick but is still spreadable.

2. Fresh labneh will keep for 3–4 days in an airtight container in the refrigerator, and for up to 2 weeks if rolled into balls and submerged in olive oil.

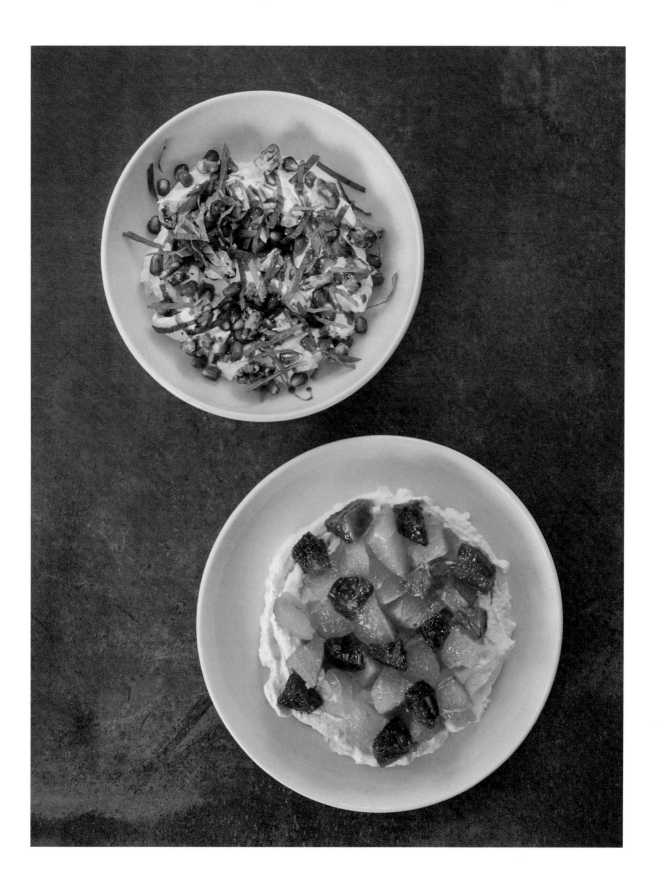

This easy recipe is originally from Pennsylvania. When I was at Barr Camp (see p. 141), Zach Miller cooked something similar for his visiting friends and it was delicious. It's great served straight from the oven with cold milk, or you can cut it into squares and take it with you out on a run.

BAKED OATMEAL

SERVES 6

240g (8½oz) whole rolled oats

60g (2⅓oz) unsalted butter, melted and slightly cooled

1 banana, mashed

150g (5oz) mixed dried berries (such as blueberries, cranberries, lingonberries or raisins)

2 large (US extra large) eggs, beaten

420ml (generous 1⅔ cups) milk (dairy or non-dairy)

120ml (½ cup) honey

1 tsp baking powder

1 tsp ground cinnamon

¼ tsp salt

1. Preheat the oven to 180°C/350°F/Gas 4 and line a large baking dish (about 32 x 25cm/13 x 10in) with greaseproof paper.

2. Mix all the ingredients together in a large bowl until well combined, then pour into the prepared baking dish.

3. Bake for 35 minutes, or until the mixture has just set. Allow to cool in the dish for 5 minutes before serving.

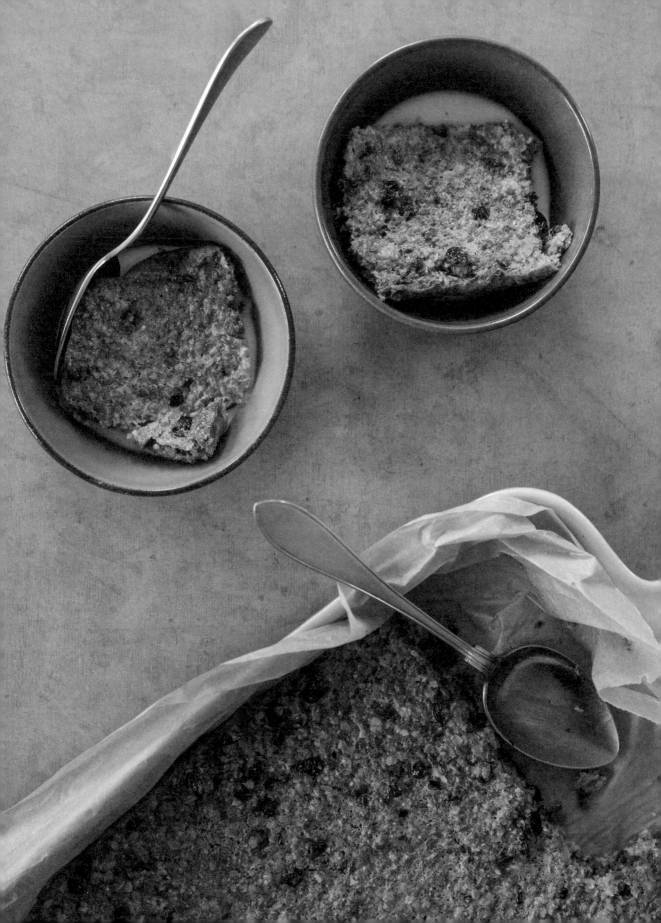

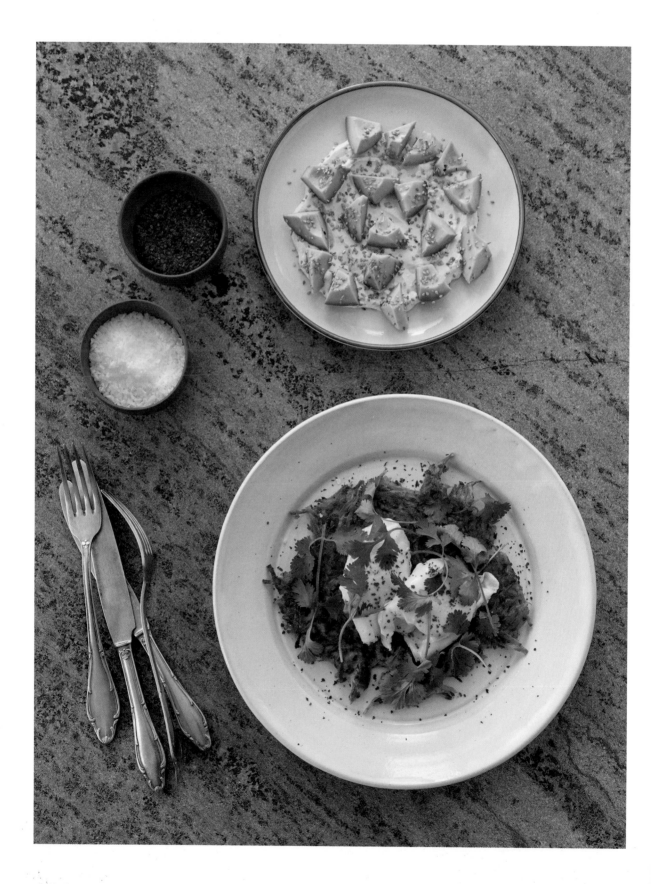

This is perfect after a weekend long run! The sweet potatoes are rich in slow-burning carbohydrates – just what you need to replenish your energy stores. The eggs are high in good cholesterol and protein – both necessary for good recovery.

SWEET POTATO ROSTI WITH POACHED EGGS

SERVES 4

1 tsp white wine vinegar

8 eggs

a handful of fresh coriander, (cilantro) picked, to serve

a pinch of Turkish dried chilli flakes (pul biber), to taste (optional)

FOR THE ROSTIS:

2 sweet potatoes, peeled and coarsely grated

a bunch of spring onions (scallions), finely sliced

1 tsp salt

1 tsp ground coriander

1 tsp ground cumin

1 tbsp plain flour

1 egg

olive oil, for cooking

freshly ground black pepper, to taste

1. Preheat the oven to 140°C/275°F/Gas 1.

2. To make the rostis, mix the potatoes, onions and salt in a bowl and allow to stand for 15 minutes, for the salt to draw out excess water. Drain in a sieve and try to press out as much liquid as you can. Transfer to a mixing bowl and add the spices, flour and a few grindings of black pepper and stir until the mixture is evenly coated. Crack in the egg and mix well.

3. Heat a frying pan over a medium heat and drizzle in enough olive oil to coat the bottom of the pan. Carefully spoon in a quarter of the rosti mixture, press into flat patties and cook for 6–8 minutes, or until the underside is crisp. Use 2 fish slices to flip the rosti over and cook for a further 4–5 minutes on the other side or until crisp and golden brown. Transfer to a baking tray and keep warm in the oven while you fry the remaining rostis.

4. For the poached eggs, bring a large saucepan of water to a simmer and add the vinegar. Crack 3 eggs into 3 separate cups (this makes it easier to get the eggs into the water). Gently swirl the water with a whisk to create a whirlpool, then gently pour the eggs into the centre, one after another (don't poach more than 3 eggs at a time or the water cools too much). Cook for 3 minutes, if you like them soft in the middle, then remove with a slotted spoon to drain on kitchen paper. Repeat until all the eggs are cooked.

5. Serve each rosti topped with 2 poached eggs, fresh coriander and a pinch of chilli flakes (if using).

This is hardly a recipe at all, but it's a nice simple side dish to have when getting back from a weekend morning run or when enjoying a day off!

TAHINI YOGURT WITH AVOCADO AND SESAME

SERVES 4 (PICTURED ON P.28)

2 ripe avocados, halved and pitted
extra-virgin olive oil, to taste
2 tbsp toasted sesame seeds
sea salt, to taste

FOR THE TAHINI YOGURT:
200g (7oz) Greek yogurt
2 tbsp tahini, or to taste
extra-virgin olive oil, to taste
1 small garlic clove, crushed (optional)
sea salt, to taste

1. For the tahini yogurt, mix the yogurt in a bowl with the tahini, a generous dash of olive oil and a pinch of salt. Taste to see whether you think it needs more tahini – it should taste as strong or as mild as you like. If using, you can also add a touch of crushed garlic at this point.

2. You can serve this individually or as a dip to share, so spread the tahini yogurt over serving plates or a platter as necessary.

3. Scoop the flesh from the avocado skins, cut it into bite-size pieces and arrange on top of the yogurt. Drizzle over some more olive oil and a scattering of toasted sesame seeds and finish with another pinch of salt.

The texture of chia pudding does take a little bit of getting used to at first, but it's worth persevering as it's a great vehicle for other delicious flavours, such as the coconut and peach in this recipe. The list of health benefits attributed to chia seeds seems to be almost endless – for runners it's usefully high in iron, a nutrient that long-distance runners often struggle to get enough of in their diets, and calcium, which is essential for maintaining strong bone structure.

COCONUT CHIA PUDDING WITH WHITE PEACH AND POMEGRANATE

SERVES 4

60g (2¹/₃oz) chia seeds
1 x 400ml (1²/₃ cups) can coconut milk
1 tbsp honey, or more to taste
a pinch of salt

TO SERVE:
2 ripe white peaches, pitted and chopped into bite-size pieces
seeds of ½ pomegranate
4 tsp flax seeds

1. Put the chia seeds into a bowl. Whisk together the coconut milk, honey and salt, pour the mixture over the chia and mix well. Allow to stand for at least 20 minutes until the mixture has thickened. Alternatively, store in the refrigerator overnight, covered.

2. When ready to eat, stir the pudding and divide it between serving bowls. Serve topped with the peach chunks, pomegranate and flax seeds.

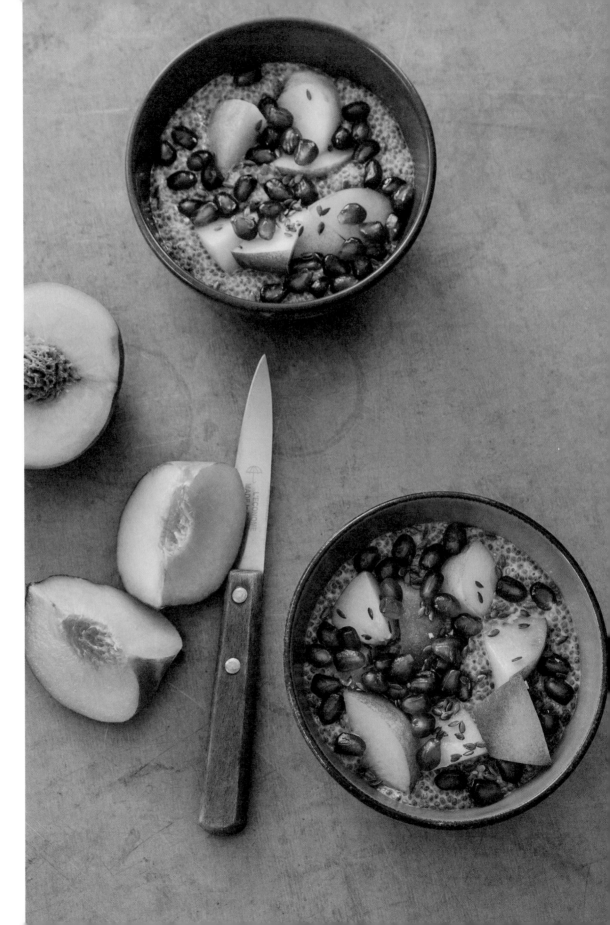

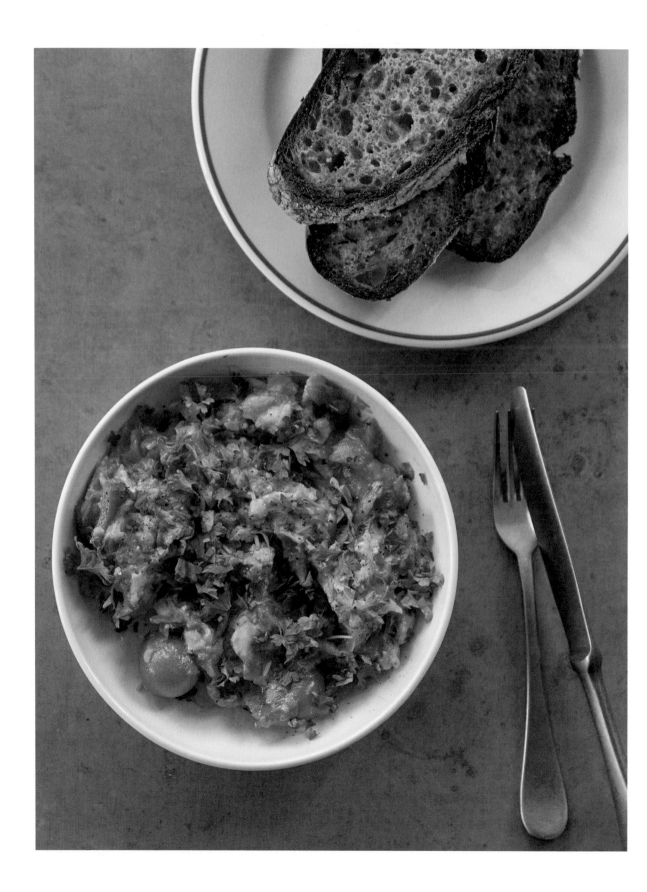

Menemen is a Turkish breakfast dish, although it makes a great
light lunch, too.

'MENEMEN' TURKISH SCRAMBLED EGGS WITH LEEK AND RED PEPPERS

SERVES 4

2 tbsp olive oil

1 leek, cleaned and chopped

1 red pepper, deseeded and finely
    chopped

2 garlic cloves, crushed

a pinch of dried chilli flakes

20 cherry tomatoes

6 eggs, beaten

a handful of chopped flat-leaf parsley

sea salt and freshly ground black
    pepper, to taste

toast, warm flatbreads, crumbled
    feta cheese or Turkish yogurt, to
    serve

1. Heat the olive oil in a frying pan over a medium heat, add the leek and red pepper and season with salt and pepper. Cook, stirring regularly, for 5 minutes until the vegetables are softened, turning down the heat if they begin to colour too much. Add the garlic, chilli flakes and tomatoes and cook for a further 5 minutes until the tomatoes begin to burst. The mixture shouldn't be too wet, so cook until most of the tomato liquid has evaporated.

2. Season the beaten eggs with salt and pepper and pour into the pan. Cook over a gentle heat, stirring all the time, until just set. Sprinkle over the chopped parsley and serve immediately.

3. This is great with toast, warm flatbreads, crumbled feta cheese or Turkish yogurt.

Steak and eggs feels like the ultimate old-fashioned American breakfast; a plate of pure protein and fat. Both ingredients are high in protein and the steak contains plenty of iron and vitamins B12 and B6 – three micronutrients that endurance runners often struggle to get enough of in their diet. The eggs are high in vitamin D, which helps the body absorb calcium. Add some purple sprouting broccoli and fresh jalapeños for a bit of a kick.

STEAK AND EGGS WITH PURPLE SPROUTING BROCCOLI AND JALAPEÑOS

SERVES 4

2 x 200g (7oz) grass-fed ribeye steaks (at room temperature)

olive oil, for cooking

1 garlic clove, smashed

1 large onion, finely chopped

3 medium potatoes (about 300g /11oz), peeled and chopped into 1–2cm (½–¾in) pieces

a pat of butter

4 eggs

350g (12oz) purple sprouting broccoli, stalks trimmed

a bunch of spring onions (scallions), thinly sliced

a bunch of fresh coriander (cilantro), leaves, picked and coarsely chopped

2 fresh jalapeños, sliced (deseeded, depending on whether you like it hot!)

sea salt and freshly ground black pepper, to taste

1. Season the steaks with salt and pepper.

2. Heat a glug of olive oil in a large frying pan over a medium heat, add the garlic and cook until it just starts to colour, then add the onion and sweat for 2–3 minutes until it begins to soften. Add the potatoes and a pinch of salt, reduce the heat and sauté for about 20 minutes, stirring occasionally, until the potatoes are cooked through and golden brown all over.

3. Meanwhile, heat another frying pan until smoking hot. Add a little oil and the steaks, then add half of the butter and lift the steaks so that the butter runs underneath. Cook for 1 minute, then reduce the heat and cook for 4–5 minutes. Turn the steaks, add the remaining butter and cook for a further 3–4 minutes. Depending on the thickness of the steaks, this should leave the meat a little pink in the middle. Adjust cooking times for more or less well-done. Remove the steaks from the pan and leave them to rest for 5 minutes.

4. Wipe the pan clean with kitchen paper and add a little more olive oil. Crack in the eggs and fry over a medium heat until cooked to your liking, then remove and set aside. Add the broccoli and fry for 3–4 minutes until the stalks are slightly tender and the florets are charred.

5. To serve, divide the potatoes among 4 plates. Slice the steak into thin slices and place on top of the potatoes. Add an egg and some broccoli to each plate and finish with a sprinkling of spring onions, fresh coriander and as much jalapeño as you can handle.

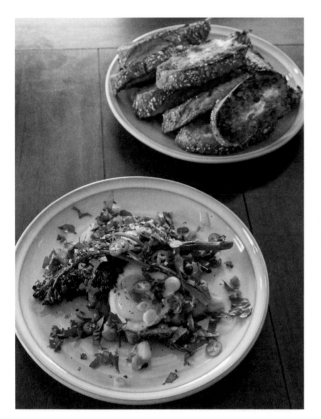

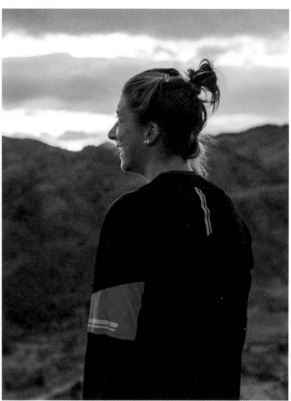

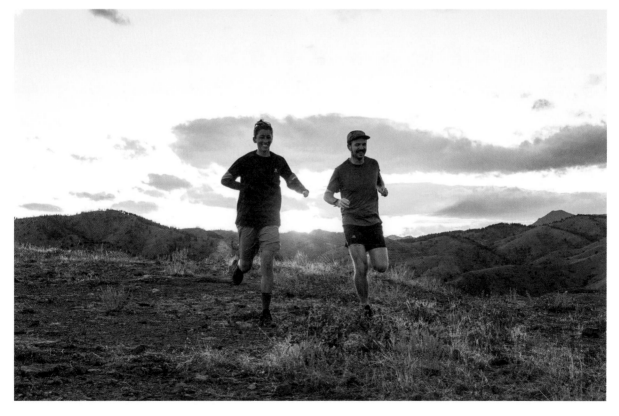

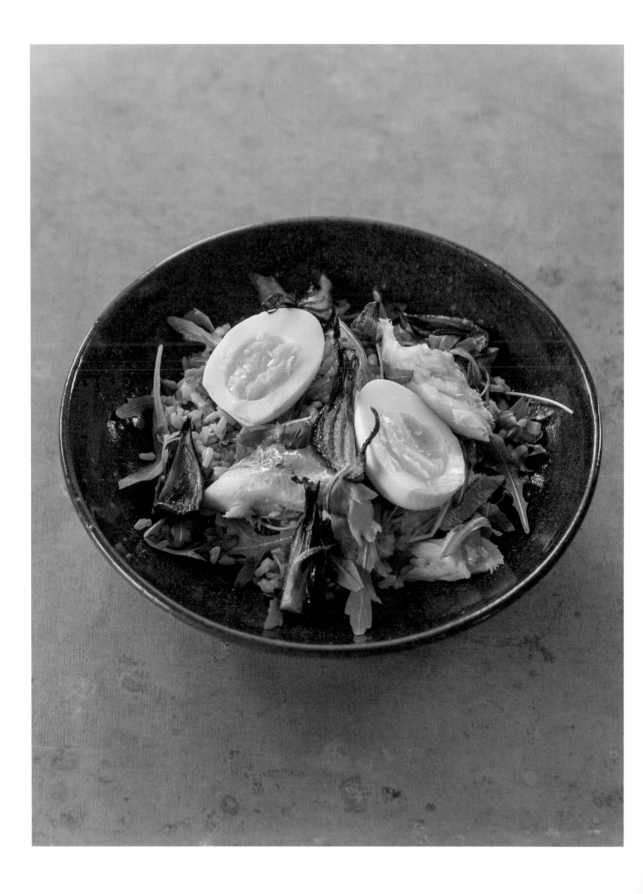

This classic British breakfast dish is traditionally made with smoked haddock. In Sweden, smoked haddock is hard to get hold of, so I've replaced it with smoked mackerel, which I think works just as well. The heavier smoking that mackerel generally gets stands up well to the strong flavours of the dish. If you struggle to imagine eating curry and smoked fish for breakfast, it works just as well for lunch or dinner.

SMOKED MACKEREL KEDGEREE

SERVES 4

3 red onions, cut into wedges

a drizzle of olive oil

200g (7oz) brown rice

4 eggs

1 tbsp butter

2 tsp curry powder (as hot as you like)

1 yellow onion, finely diced

4 smoked mackerel fillets, broken into bite-size pieces, bones removed

2 handfuls of rocket (arugula)

sea salt and freshly ground black pepper, to taste

1. Preheat the oven to 180°C/350°F/Gas 4.

2. Put the red onion wedges into a roasting pan and toss with olive oil and a pinch of salt. Roast for about 20 minutes until golden and cooked through.

3. Meanwhile, cook the brown rice according to the packet instructions, then drain and set aside.

4. Place the eggs in a saucepan of cold water and bring to the boil, then reduce to a simmer and cook for 6 minutes. Drain and briefly hold under cold running water until just cool enough to handle, then peel.

5. In a large frying pan, heat the butter over a medium heat until bubbling, then add the curry powder and cook for 1 minute. Add the diced onion, reduce the heat and cook for 10 minutes, stirring occasionally, until translucent but not coloured. Add the cooked rice to the pan, increase the heat to high and cook, stirring constantly, for 3–4 minutes until all the rice is golden. Season with salt and pepper, then add the roasted onions and smoked mackerel, gently stirring so as to not break up the fish, and cook for a final 2 minutes.

6. To serve, stir in the rocket and divide the mixture. Cut the boiled eggs in half and place on top of each serving.

If you ever go up to Barr Camp, these pancakes are what you'll be served for breakfast. Easy to prepare and nutritious, they keep you going for a big day on the mountain.

NEAL'S PIKES PEAK POWER PANCAKES

SERVES 4-6 HUNGRY CAMPERS

130g (4½oz or 1 cup) plain flour

35g (1¹/₅oz or ¼ cup) buckwheat flour

35g (1¹/₅oz or ¼ cup) wholewheat flour

40g (1³/₅oz or ¼ cup) polenta or medium-ground cornmeal

25g (1oz or ¼ cup) rolled oats

2 tbsp brown sugar

2 tbsp unsweetened cocoa powder

1 tbsp baking powder

¼ tsp bicarbonate of soda

1 tsp ground cinnamon

¼ tsp ground nutmeg

½ tsp vanilla extract

½ apple, finely diced

4 tbsp apple sauce or juice

milk or water, as needed

neutral oil, for frying

TO SERVE (OPTIONAL):

nut butter

maple syrup

a handful of walnuts, pecans or almonds, chopped

1. Combine the dry ingredients in a large bowl and mix until well combined. Stir in the vanilla, diced apple and apple sauce or juice until well combined, then whisk in enough milk or water to bring the mixture to a thick yet pourable consistency.

2. Heat a frying pan or cast-iron skillet over a medium heat, add a little oil to the pan, then ladle in enough batter to form a pancake (about 3–4 tablespoons). Swirl the pan a little to spread evenly. Cook for about 3 minutes until bubbles break the surface of the pancake and the underside is golden brown. Flip with a spatula and cook for a further 1 minute on the other side. Remove from the pan to a plate.

3. Repeat until all the batter is used up.

4. Serve as you wish, perhaps spread with some nut butter or with a drizzle of maple syrup and a scattering of chopped nuts.

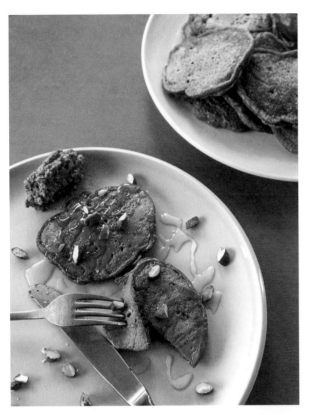
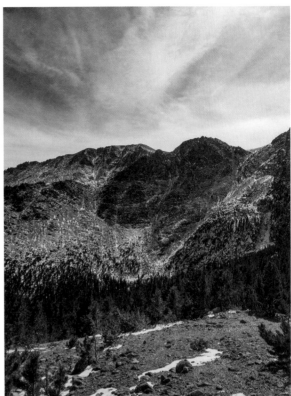
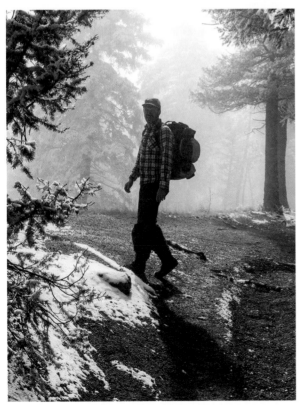
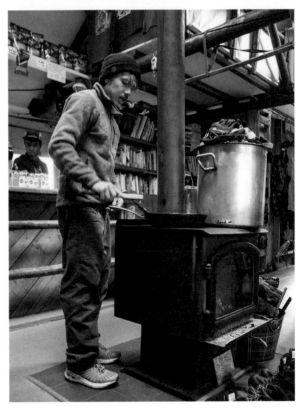

On the Trail with:

Courtney Dauwalter

Colorado, USA

IT WAS WITH SOME nervousness that I hurriedly drove north to Golden, on the outskirts of Denver, for a lunch run with Courtney Dauwalter. A snowstorm was forecast and I didn't want to miss out on the chance to run with this legend of the trail-running world.

A former science teacher from Minnesota, Courtney Dauwalter spent her youth cross-country running and skiing, eventually reaching State Champion status in Nordic skiing through hard work and many dark mornings training before school, and winning a scholarship to the university of Denver. Growing up in a family with older brothers, she clearly had a competitive streak from the get-go.

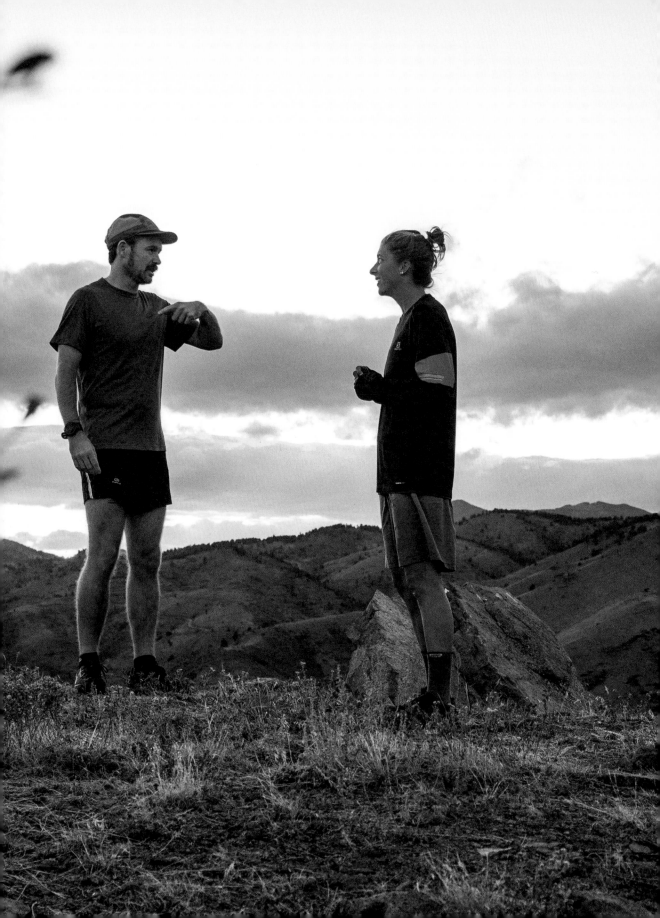

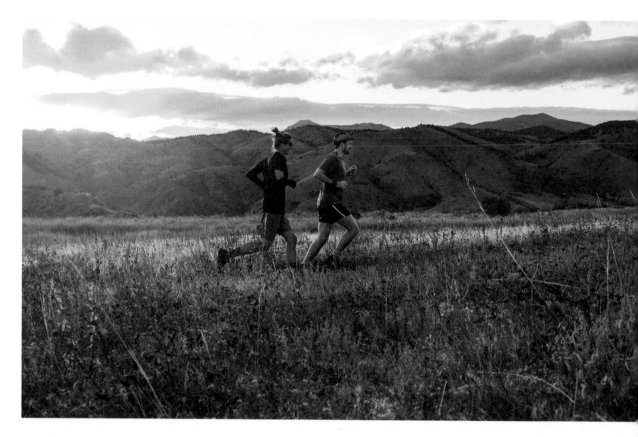

Race stats (selected)

2017 Moab 240 Endurance Run: 1st overall
2017 Soochow International Ultra-Marathon 24 Hour Race: 1st female (159.3 miles)
2018 Western States 100: 1st female
2018 Ultra-Trail Mt. Fuji 100: 1st female
2018 Tahoe 200: 1st female
2019 Miut 120km Madeira Island Ultra Trail: 1st female

She kept running after college, but cites the DNF (did not finish) in her first 100-mile (160km) race, Run Rabbit Run in 2012, as the turning moment in her running career. Since then, her performances have been consistently amazing. Flying some-what under the radar of the mainstream sports media, she was winning numerous titles, from 50K (31-mile) trails, to 100-mile (160km) mountain races, to 24-hour endurance feats, but it wasn't until she won the Moab 240 Endurance Run (yes, 240 miles /386km!) outright in 2017, beating the second-place finisher by almost 10 hours, that the world sat up and took notice. It was a performance that stopped the long-distance running community in its tracks!

2018 was a big year for Courtney, who won almost every race she entered, including the Sean O'Brien 100K, the Western States 100, the Ultra-Trail Mt. Fuji and the Tahoe 200, where she led the race overall until mile 196 (315km) and beat the third-placed runner by more than 10 hours, and led to her winning the prestigious Ultra Runner of the Year award.

I was lucky with the weather and arrived in good time to meet Courtney and her husband Kevin, also a keen trail runner, just outside the city. We headed off to run a few gentle miles in what she describes as her 'door-step trails'. She lives in an ideal location; a mere mile or so from her front door lie hundreds of miles of trails into the foothills of the Rockies and the views are spectacular.

It was great to hear some of Courtney's stories from the trails. In particular, her exhaustion-induced hallucinations are hilarious and it was fascinating to hear how she finds the inner strength to dig deep when the going gets hard. It's clear from her race results (and the type of races that she excels in) that mental toughness is one of her major strengths, but it's the smile on Courtney's face the whole time we are on the trail that testifies to the fact that running means so much more to her than just winning races. Courtney is undoubtably one of the toughest athletes in the sport, but she does it with such humour and humility, it's truly inspirational.

After the run, we headed to a local brewery on the outskirts of town, which was full of people enjoying a post-run or mountain-biker's beer. With a late-autumn chill in the air, it was brown ales for everyone. We agreed that I would make breakfast the following morning. Later that evening, the predicted snow storm arrived, and I had another nervous drive heading over to Courtney's house in knee-deep snow the next day.

I couldn't resist making steak and eggs for breakfast. It's a classic diner breakfast, but I add purple sprouting broccoli, plenty of fresh green chilli and fresh coriander (cilantro) to give it a healthier and lighter touch (see recipe on p.34).

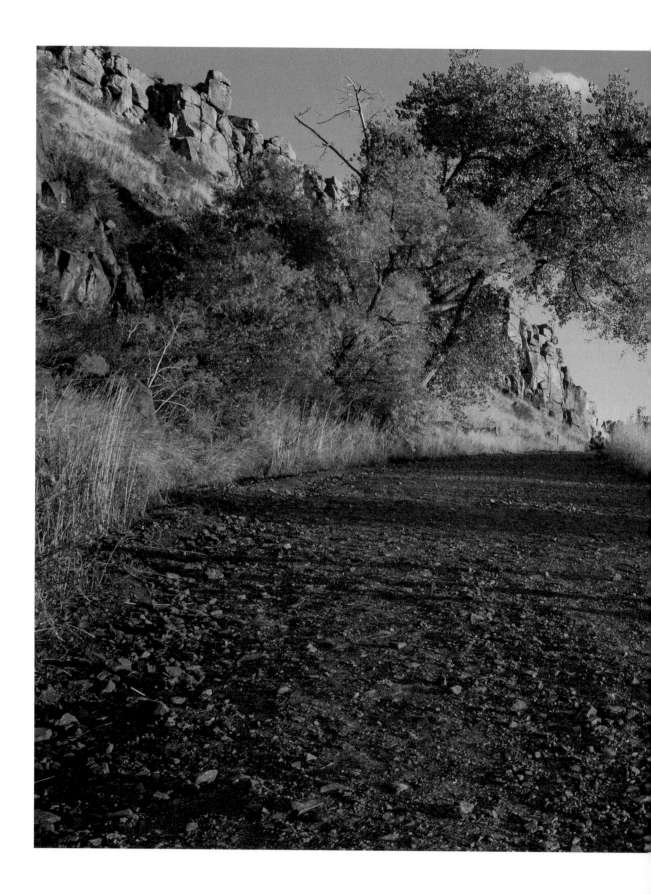

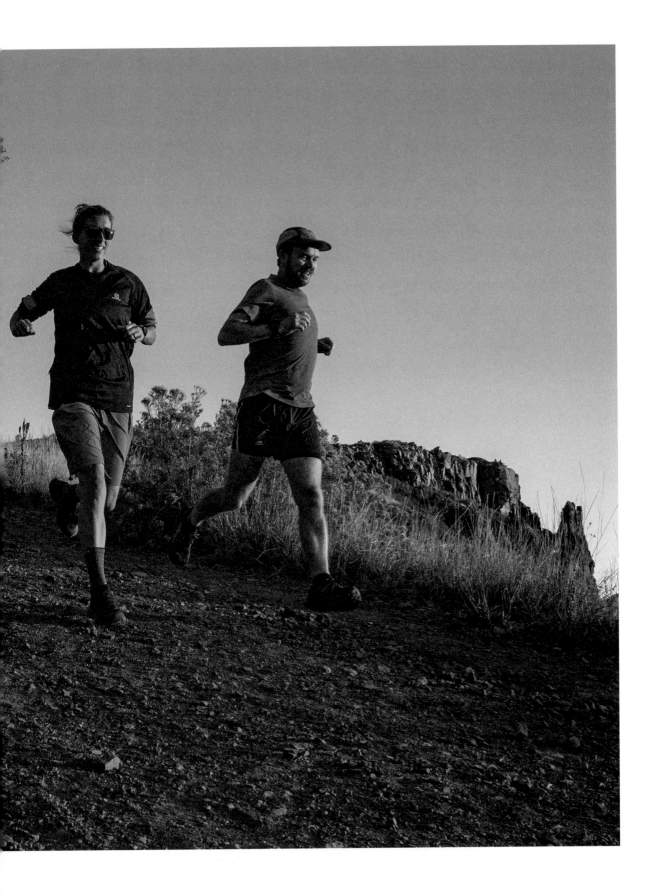

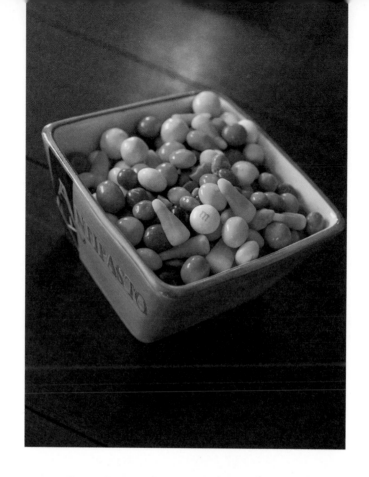

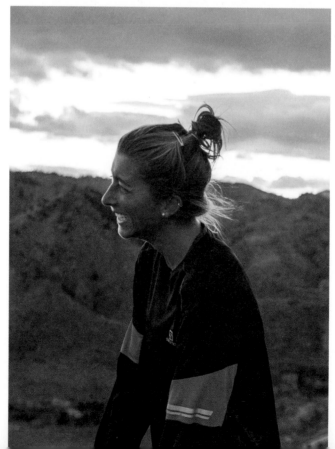

«If you have to turn back after a mile because your body says 'no', do it»

After being a vegetarian for 13 years, Courtney does now eat meat again, so I picked a couple of lovely grass-fed ribeye steaks and served them with a few slices of toasted seeded sourdough loaf from a local bakery. Courtney meanwhile provided the biggest cup of coffee I've ever had! It went down well – a small amount of protein and carbs from the potatoes are good pre-run, although the fresh green chillies are optional just before exercising!

I found out that the night before the Tahoe 200, she ate candy corn and pizza, and after the race refuelled on nachos loaded with cheese and barbecue chicken and drank plenty of beer. It's a good example of how, when it comes to food, Courtney has no fixed plan. She listens to her body, eats what she feels like, when she feels like it, and takes this approach into her training schedule, too. While she generally averages between 100–110 miles (160–177km) per week, she doesn't do any specific speed sessions or hill training. Instead, she just listens to her body and pushes when it feels good, holding back when it doesn't: 'If you have to turn back after a mile because your body says "no", do it. There's no need to struggle on and potentially injure yourself.'

When I met Courtney, she was tapering before heading to Tennessee, to run the Big's Backyard Ultra, a loop of 4.15 miles (6.68km), restarted every hour until there is only one runner left. Courtney finished second place after running 279 miles (449km) in just under three days. For the race, she ate 'Honey Stinger' waffles, cheese quesadillas, pierogis and pancakes for the first 30 hours, and then opted for McDonald's double cheeseburgers with extra pickles thereafter. When running these sort of distances, eating what you feel like and what you crave is probably what your body needs most. There is no point trying to force down handfuls of trail mix if you are really struggling to eat it. Likewise, if you are sick and tired of gels, take a break from them and have a salty snack from the aid station.

I couldn't fail to be impressed by Courtney. Although, in her unassuming way, she feels uncomfortable being seen as a role model, her demeanour out on the trails is a testament to her. Even 40 hours into a gruelling race, in the midst of hallucinations and struggling to keep food down, she still has the grace to thank the aid-station workers for being there and pose for a few selfies with young fans. A smile is never far from her face, even in the depths of mid-race misery. For her, it's all about the joy of just being out there on the trails, whether it's alone or with friends. •

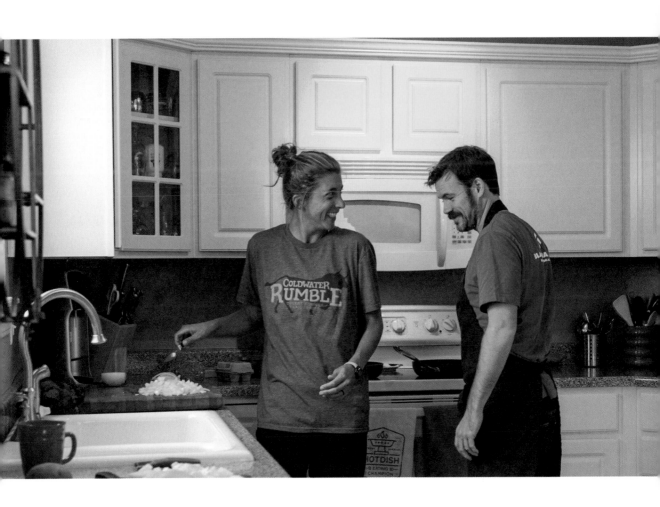

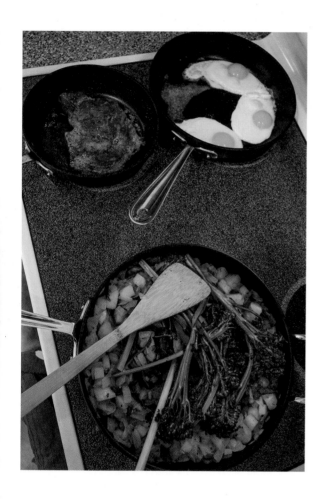

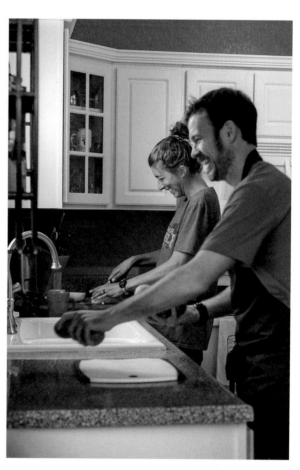

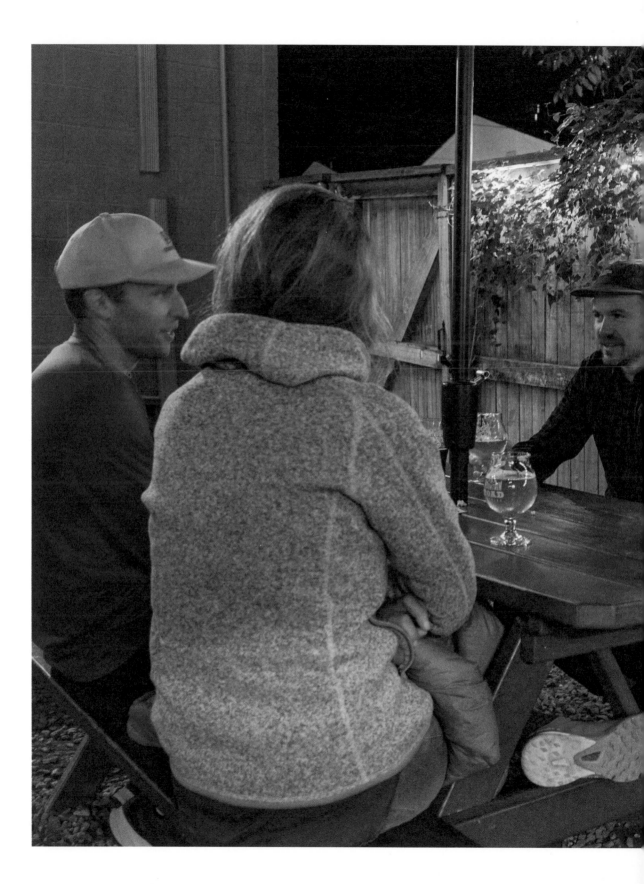

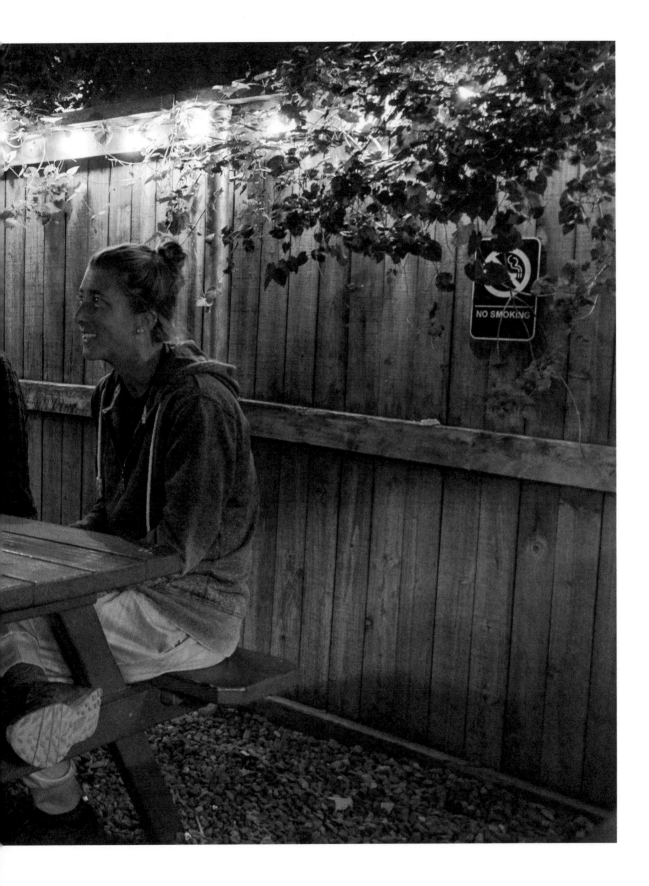

CHAPTER TWO

Snacks and Light Lunches

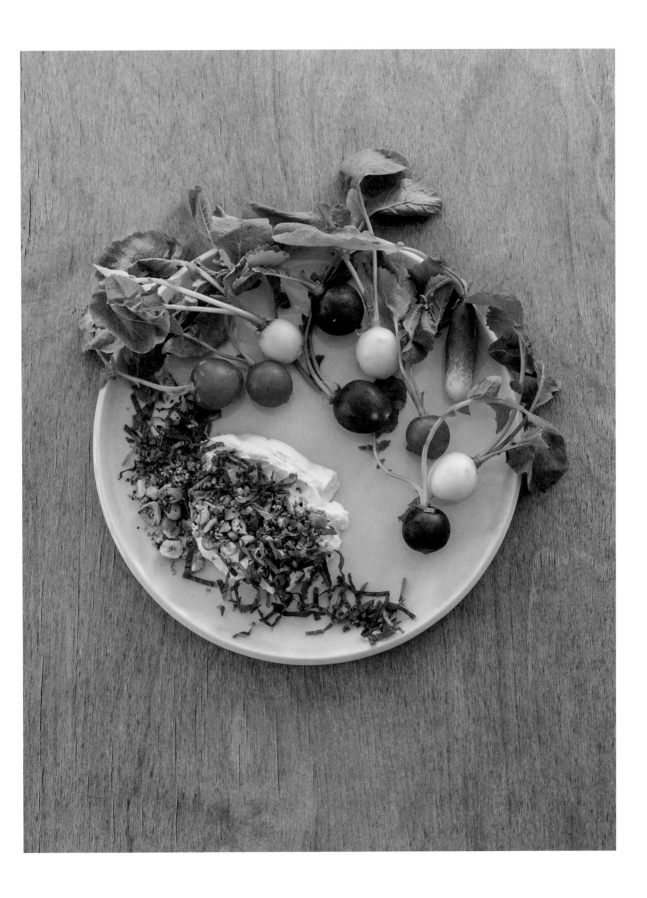

This only takes a few minutes to prepare and is great as a pre-dinner snack or if you need something quick after an afternoon training run.

RADISHES, LABNEH AND HAZELNUT DUKKAH

SERVES 4

24 mixed radishes, cleaned, with leaves untrimmed
400g (14oz) Labneh (see p.24)
a handful of mint, coarsely chopped

FOR THE HAZELNUT DUKKAH:
1 tsp toasted coriander seeds
1 tsp toasted cumin seeds
½ tsp dried chilli flakes
½ tsp sea salt
200g (7oz) roasted hazelnuts

1. To make the dukkah, pulse the coriander and cumin seeds, chilli flakes and salt in a food processor until they have broken up a bit, then add the roasted hazelnuts and pulse again, until they are roughly broken up. It's nice to keep some texture, otherwise it can be like eating dust. Dukkah will keep for months in a jar, so it's always worth making more than you need.

2. Either divide the radishes and labneh among 4 serving plates or serve on 1 large platter. Sprinkle the dukkah and chopped mint over the top of the labneh. To eat, dip a radish into the labneh, ensuring you get a good amount of the dukkah and mint at the same time.

Beetroot borani is a Iranian yogurt dip.

BEETROOT BORANI WITH FLATBREADS

SERVES 4

300g (11oz) cooked and peeled beetroot
300g (11oz) full-fat Greek yogurt
1 garlic clove, crushed
2 tbsp red wine vinegar
4 tbsp extra-virgin olive oil, plus extra for drizzling
a few dill sprigs, chopped, plus extra to garnish
100g (3¾oz) feta cheese, crumbled
50g (2oz) chopped toasted almonds
sea salt, to taste
wholewheat flatbreads or pitta, toasted, to serve

1. Blend the beetroot to a coarse purée in a food processor – you want some texture so don't overblend. Transfer to a bowl, add the yogurt, garlic, vinegar, oil, dill and a pinch of salt and mix until well combined. Check the seasoning and adjust if needed.

2. Spread the beetroot purée on a serving plate and sprinkle over the feta, almonds and extra dill sprigs, then drizzle with a little olive oil. Serve with toasted wholemeal flatbreads or pitta on the side for dipping.

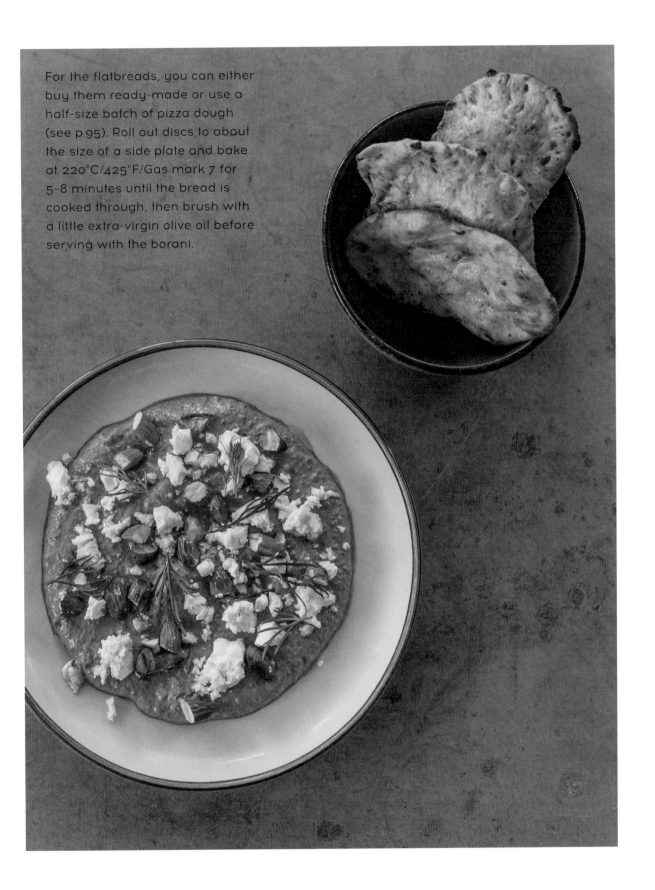

For the flatbreads, you can either buy them ready-made or use a half-size batch of pizza dough (see p.95). Roll out discs to about the size of a side plate and bake at 220°C/425°F/Gas mark 7 for 5–8 minutes until the bread is cooked through, then brush with a little extra-virgin olive oil before serving with the borani.

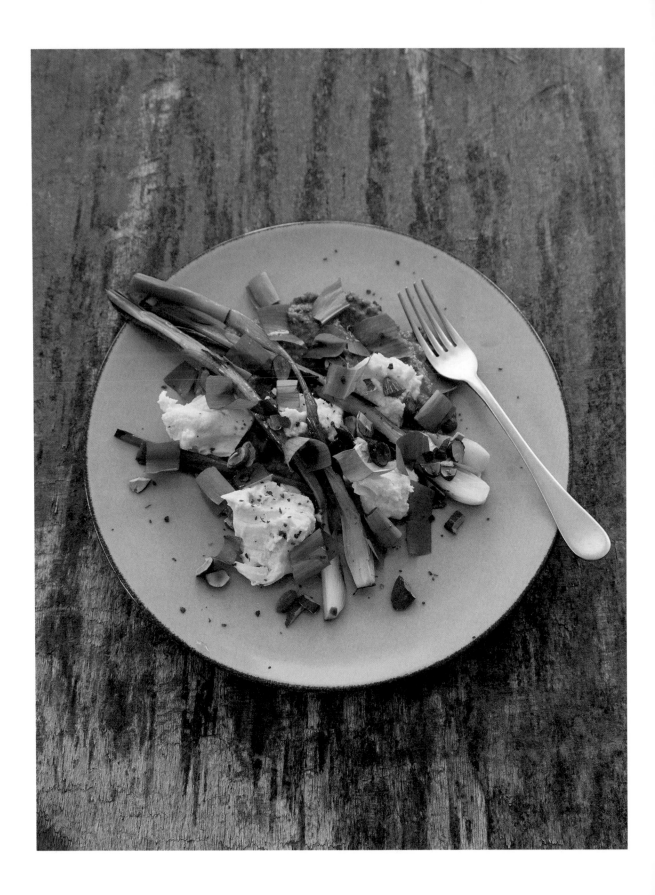

Romesco and grilled spring onions (scallions) is a classic Catalan combination. Traditionally, calçots (a cross between a spring onion and a leek) are traditionally grilled over the fire, torn apart and dipped into romesco sauce – a very messy but delicious celebration of the beginning of spring. With the addition of buffalo mozzarella, it becomes a great light lunch.

ROMESCO WITH BUFFALO MOZARELLA, CHARRED SPRING ONIONS AND WILD GARLIC

SERVES 4

2 large roasted red peppers, peeled and deseeded (you can use good-quality ones from a jar)

200g (7oz) toasted skin-on almonds

1 garlic clove

2 tbsp red wine vinegar, or to taste

1 tsp smoked paprika, or to taste

½ tsp cayenne pepper, or to taste

100ml (scant ½ cup) extra-virgin olive oil

12 spring onions (scallions), trimmed

2 x 100g (3¾oz) buffalo mozzarella balls, torn into bite-size pieces

a handful of wild garlic (or rocket/arugula), chopped

salt and freshly ground black pepper, to taste

1. Put the peppers, three-quarters of the almonds, garlic, red wine vinegar, smoked paprika and cayenne pepper into a food processor and process until just becoming smooth. With the motor still running, slowly pour in almost all of the olive oil through the feed tube, blending until everything has come together into a thick sauce. Season with salt and pepper. Taste – you may want to add a bit more vinegar or spices. If so, add as you wish and process briefly to combine.

2. Heat a dry cast-iron frying pan until it is smoking hot, then add the spring onions and gently move them around the pan until they are evenly charred and slightly softened, about 2 minutes. Remove from the pan and drizzle with the remaining olive oil and a pinch of salt.

3. To serve, divide the romesco between 4 serving plates and top each one with a few pieces of mozzarella and 4 charred onions. Coarsely chop the remaining almonds and scatter over the plates, along with the wild garlic (or rocket).

It's common for nutritionists to talk about eating as many different coloured foods as possible – this recipe makes it easy. Rainbow chard is such a treat, as it's full of potassium, magnesium, vitamin C and a host of other micronutrients. Coupled with brown rice, which is a great slow-burning unprocessed carbohydrate, it makes for a very well-balanced meal.

RAINBOW CHARD, SQUASH AND BROWN RICE TORTILLA

SERVES 4

6 tbsp olive oil

400g (14oz) chard, washed, leaves separated, stalks thinly sliced

150g (5oz) squash or courgette (zucchini), cut into 1cm (²/₅in) chunks

2 garlic cloves, thinly sliced

200g (7oz) cooked brown rice

5 eggs

sea salt and freshly ground black pepper, to taste

lettuce leaves, to serve

1. Preheat the grill to high.

2. Heat 3 tablespoons of the olive oil in a saucepan over a low heat, add the chard stalks and squash or courgette and cook for 10–15 minutes until they begin to soften but not colour. Add the garlic and chard leaves, increase the heat slightly and cook for a further 5 minutes until the leaves are tender and any liquid released has evaporated. Add the cooked rice and season with salt and pepper.

3. Beat the eggs in a bowl, then stir in the chard and rice mixture.

4. In a non-stick ovenproof frying pan or well-used omelette pan, heat the remaining olive oil over a high heat, add the egg mixture and cook until the bottom has set and just started to colour. Slide a spatula underneath and flip the tortilla over, then cook for 2–3 minutes on that side.

5. Transfer the pan to the grill and gently cook for a further 5 minutes, at least 10–15cm (4–6in) away from the heat. Check the tortilla is ready by pressing on the top; it should be firm to the touch.

6. Flip the tortilla out onto a plate. It's great served with lettuce leaves.

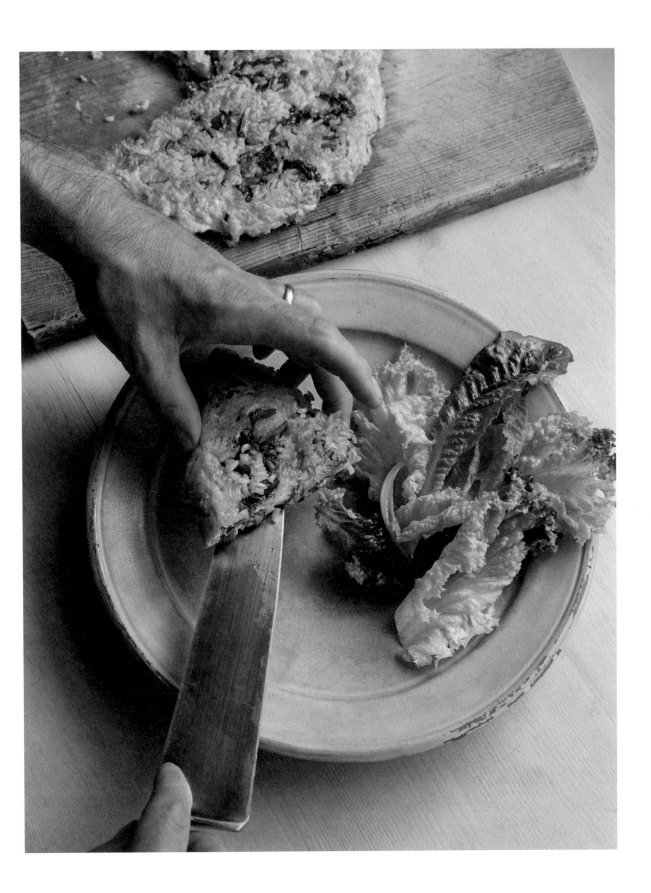

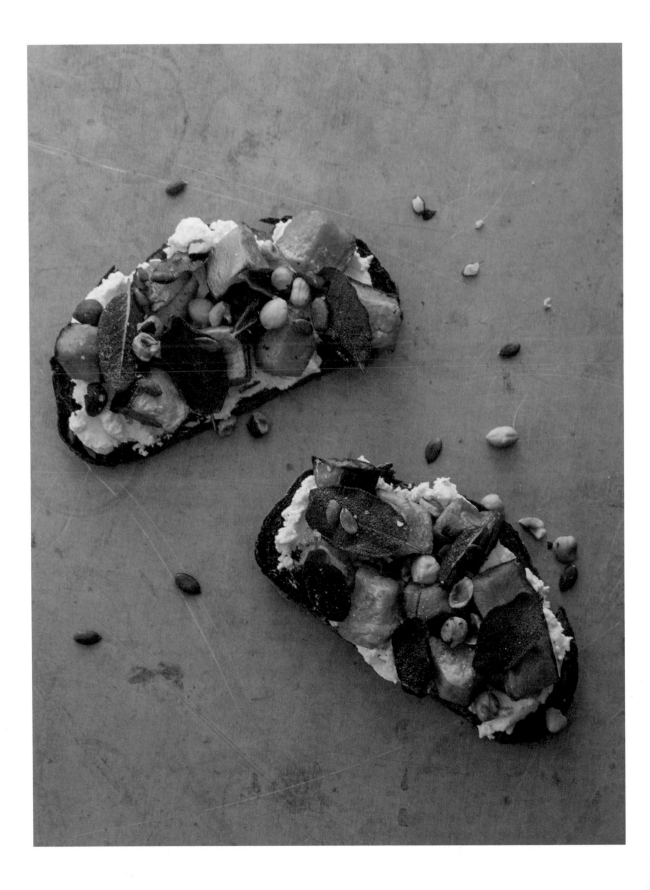

On Toast

One of the best bits about baking bread at home (see my Bread recipes on pp.182–193) is that you will always have plenty of day-old bread around, which is perfect for toasting. My Sourdough Bread, when toasted, is just as good spread with butter and homemade jam for breakfast as it is topped with fresh cheese and different roasted vegetables, as here. I love it.

GOATS' CURD, ROASTED SQUASH AND SAGE ON TOAST

SERVES 4

1kg (2¼lb) butternut squash, peeled and chopped into 2cm (¾in) chunks

extra-virgin olive oil, for drizzling

a handful of sage leaves

8 slices of Sourdough Bread (see p.185)

400g (14oz) goats' curd or fresh goats' cheese

a small handful of roasted chopped hazelnuts

2 tbsp roasted pumpkin seeds

sea salt and freshly ground black pepper, to taste

1. Preheat the oven to 180°C/350°F/Gas mark 4.

2. Place the squash in a roasting pan and season with salt, pepper and a generous glug of olive oil. Roast for 20–25 minutes until the squash is soft on the inside and golden on the outside.

3. In a small bowl, mix the sage leaves with a pinch of salt and a little olive oil until the leaves are evenly coated. Place in the roasting pan with the squash to roast for the last 3–4 minutes until they are crisp.

4. Toast the bread and spread it with the goats' curd. Arrange the roasted squash and sage leaves on the top, then sprinkle over the hazelnuts and pumpkin seeds.

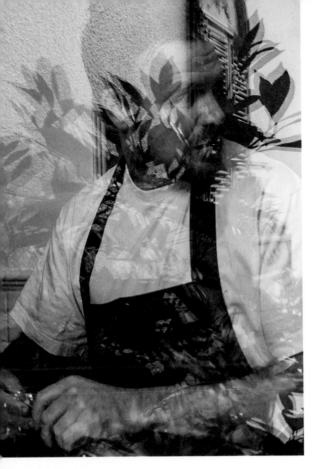

GOATS' CURD, ROAST TOMATOES AND MINT ON TOAST

SERVES 4

800g (1¾lb) ripe mixed tomatoes, halved or quartered depending on size

4 tbsp extra-virgin olive oil

2 handfuls of picked mint leaves

juice of ½ lemon

8 slices of Sourdough Bread (see p.185)

400g (14oz) goats' curd or fresh goats' cheese

sea salt, to taste

1. Preheat the oven to 160°C/325°F/Gas mark 3.

2. Put the tomatoes into a roasting tray, drizzle with half the olive oil and season with a pinch of salt. Roast for about 30 minutes until the tomatoes are soft but still hold their shape.

3. In a small bowl, dress the mint leaves with the remaining olive oil and the lemon juice and season with a pinch of salt.

4. Toast the bread and spread it with the goats' curd or cheese. Arrange the roast tomatoes on top and garnish with the dressed mint leaves.

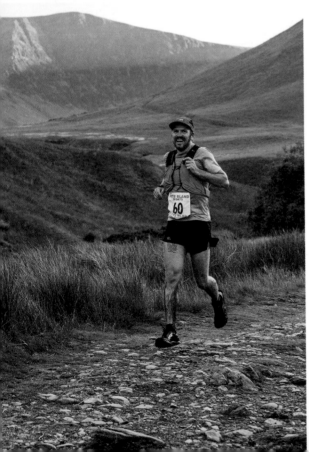

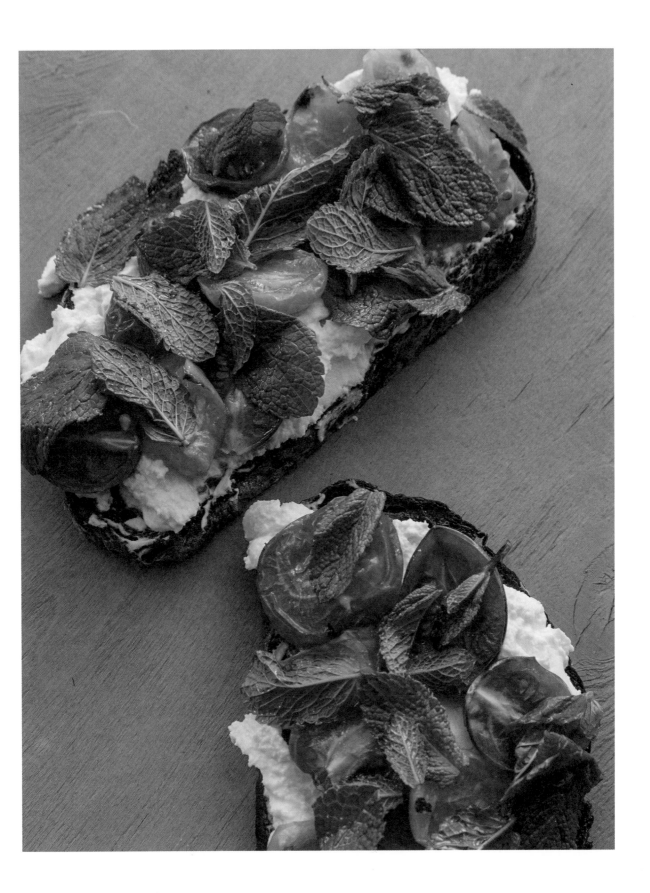

This is one of my favourites. Liver is one of the greatest sources of iron that we can eat, as is spinach; combined, you have a meal that is a real recovery boost.

DEVILLED CHICKEN LIVERS AND SPINACH ON TOAST

SERVES 4

3 tbsp plain flour

1 tsp cayenne pepper

1 tsp English mustard powder

600g (1⅓lb) chicken livers, cleaned and trimmed

3 tbsp butter

300g (11oz) spinach leaves, picked and washed

4 large slices of Sourdough Bread (see p.185)

a hearty splash of Worcestershire sauce

50ml (¼ cup) chicken stock

sea salt and freshly ground black pepper, to taste

1. In a bowl, mix together the flour, cayenne pepper and mustard with a big pinch of salt and quite a lot of pepper. Roll the chicken livers in the seasoned flour until evenly coated, then shake off any excess flour in a sieve.

2. Heat a frying pan over a high heat, add 1 tablespoon of the butter, then add the spinach. Season with a pinch of salt and pepper and cook for 2 minutes until the spinach is wilted and any liquid has evaporated.

3. Meanwhile, toast the bread, then divide the spinach among the 4 waiting pieces of toast.

4. Wipe out the frying pan and place back over a high heat. Add another 1 tablespoon of butter to the pan and, when foaming, place the chicken livers in the pan and cook for 2 minutes on each side. Add the Worcestershire sauce along with the chicken stock and bring to the boil. Remove the livers to the slices of toast.

5. Add the remaining tablespoon of butter to the pan and reduce the stock until you get a thick sauce. Pour the sauce over the livers, spinach and toast, and serve immediately.

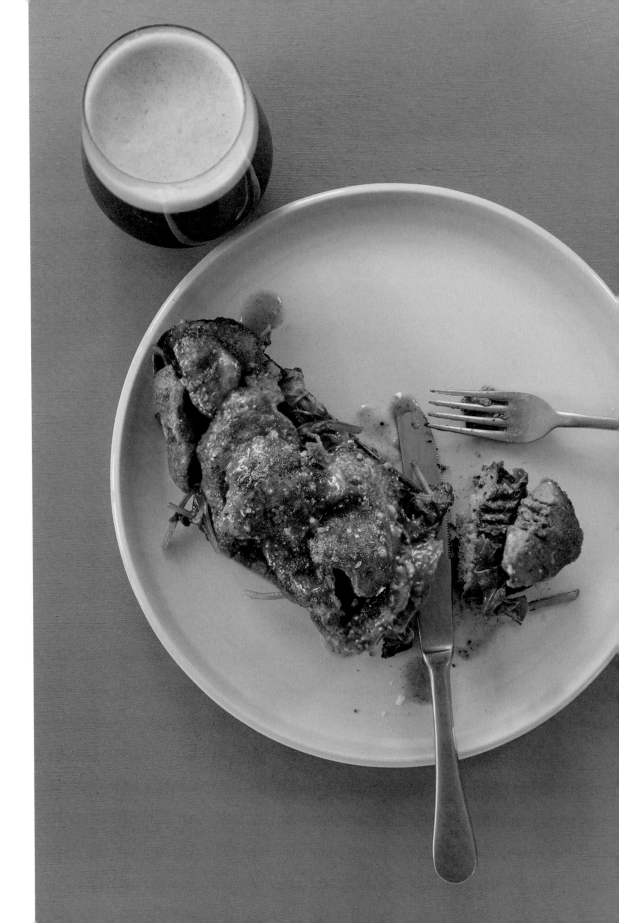

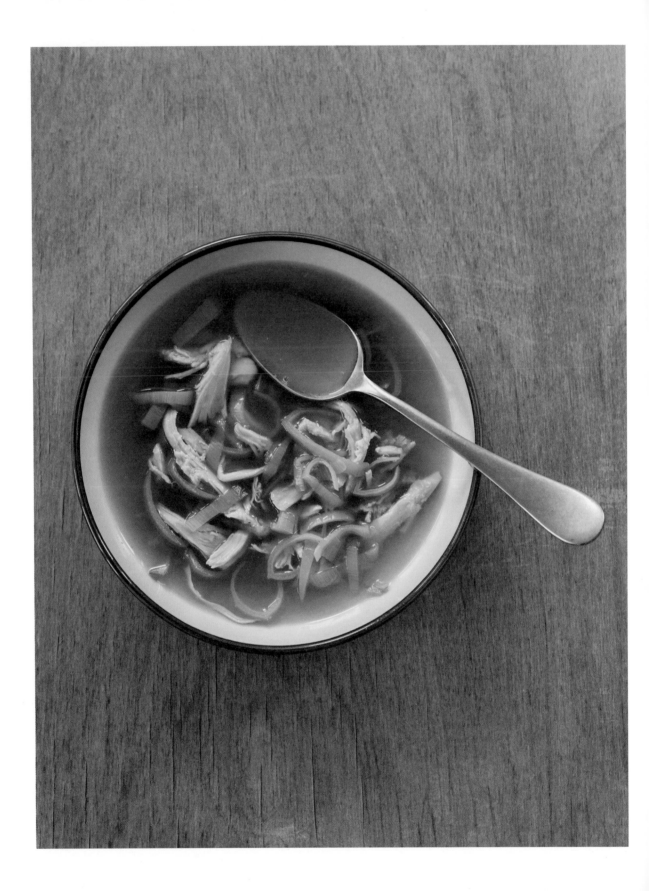

Soups and Broths

The bones from a single chicken carcass will only make enough broth for two people, so it's a good idea to save the leftover bones whenever you roast a chicken (keep them in the freezer) or ask your local butcher if they have some chicken bones you can have. The broth freezes very well, so it's always worth making extra and freezing it before the chicken meat and leeks are added.

CHICKEN AND LEEK BROTH

SERVES 4

1kg (2¼lb) chicken bones (about 2 whole carcasses)

2 garlic cloves, peeled and firmly smashed

1 onion, peeled and quartered

a pinch of salt

1 medium leek, cleaned and sliced

200g (7oz) cooked chicken (leftovers from a roast are ideal), chopped

1. Preheat the oven to 200°C/400°F/Gas 6.

2. Place the bones in a roasting tray and roast for about 30 minutes, or until golden brown. Shake the bones once or twice during cooking to make sure they colour evenly.

3. Put the roasted bones into a heavy saucepan that will fit them snugly, add the garlic and onion and pour in enough water to barely cover (about 1.5 litres /6¼ cups). Bring to a gentle simmer and simmer for 45 minutes, occasionally skimming off any foam or fat from the top (don't go overboard as the chicken fat contains a lot of flavour).

4. Strain the liquid into a new saucepan and discard the bones. Add the salt and taste. At this point, you can choose to reduce the liquid a little to deepen the flavour or keep the broth light and fresh. I often find this depends on the weather; in winter a dark, rich broth is more appealing, whereas in spring or summer you may want something lighter. Once you are happy with the taste, add the leek and bring to the boil over a medium heat. Cook for 2 minutes, then add the chicken and cook for a further 3 minutes until the leek is soft and the chicken has warmed through.

Here in Sweden, towards the end of a race they often serve hot broth – the warm savoury taste is often very welcome after a lot of sweet race food. Beef broth is rich in protein and full of other micronutrients, including potassium, magnesium and calcium, plus collagen, which yields several important amino acids. The best bones to use for this are shin bones – ask for them at your local butcher.

BEEF BROTH

SERVES 4

2kg (4½lb) beef bones, cut into 5cm (2in) chunks
4 onions, peeled and halved
2 tbsp apple cider vinegar
2 litres (8 cups) water
sea salt, to taste

1. Preheat the oven to 200°C/400°F/Gas 6.

2. Place the bones in a roasting pan and roast for about 40 minutes until dark golden brown, turning the bones twice to ensure they colour evenly.

3. Heat a cast-iron pan until smoking hot, then place the onions in the pan, cut-side down. Sear for about 3–4 minutes on all sides until the onions are quite dark in colour – this will give the broth a nice deep colour and also some sweetness.

4. Remove the bones from the oven and drain away any fat. Transfer the bones to a large saucepan, add the onion halves, vinegar and water, and bring to the boil. Reduce the heat to very low and simmer for 8–12 hours until the broth is dark and rich. From time to time, use a small ladle to skim off any fat or foam that gathers on the surface of the broth and top up with extra water as the bones become exposed.

5. Strain the broth through a fine sieve and discard the bones. Season with salt to taste. Serve immediately or cool and refrigerate. The broth will keep in the refrigerator for up to a week and also freezes well.

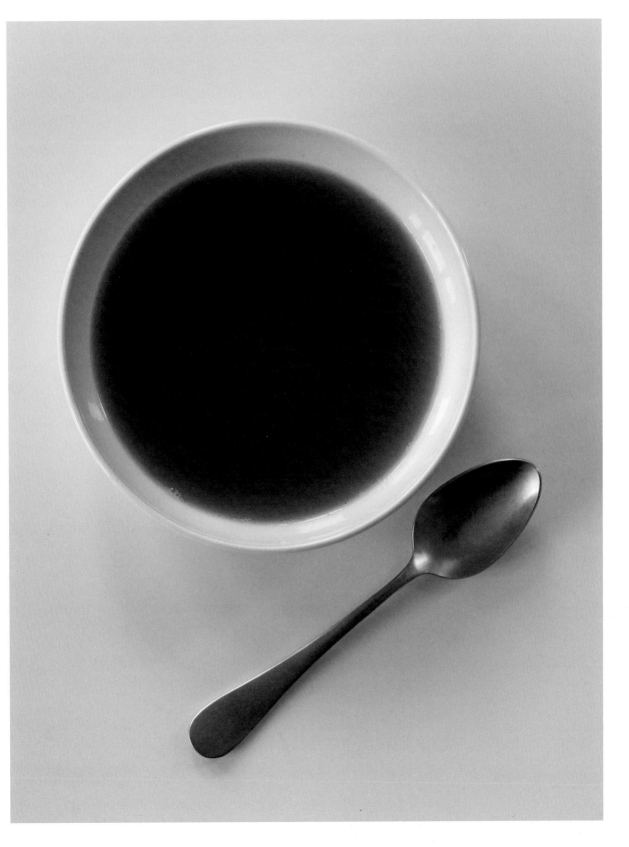

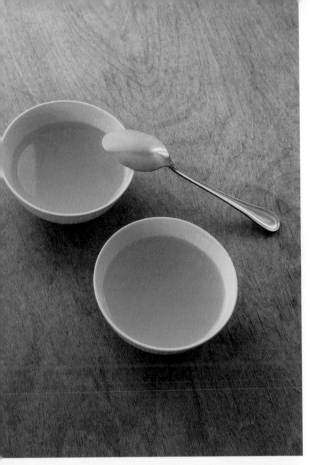

This is a good alternative to meat-based stocks and is much better than those salt-laden commercial stock (bouillon) cubes or powders. It's great to add to soups and sauces, but as a hot drink after a long cold run it's delicious!

VEGETABLE BROTH

SERVES 4 (MAKES ABOUT 1 LITRE/4 CUPS)

4 large carrots, coarsely chopped

5 celery stalks, coarsely chopped

1 fennel bulb, coarsely chopped

1 large leek, washed, trimmed and coarsely chopped

1 whole green garlic bulb, sliced widthways

5 spring onions (scallions), coarsely chopped

a small bunch each of thyme, fennel fronds and parsley, tied together with kitchen string

sea salt, to taste

1. Put all the ingredients into a large saucepan or stock pot and cover with cold water (about 1.2 litres/5 cups). Bring to the boil, then reduce to a simmer and gently cook for about 45 minutes until the vegetables are tender and cooked through but not mushy and falling apart. Strain out the vegetables and season the clear broth with salt to taste.

2. If not using immediately, it will keep in the refrigerator for 3–4 days in a sealed container, and it also freezes very well.

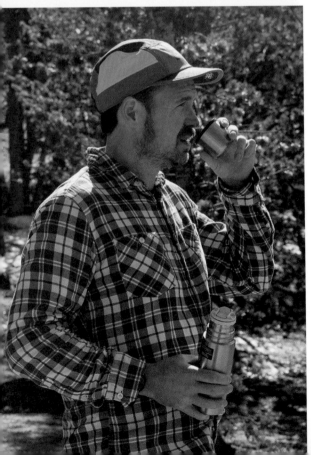

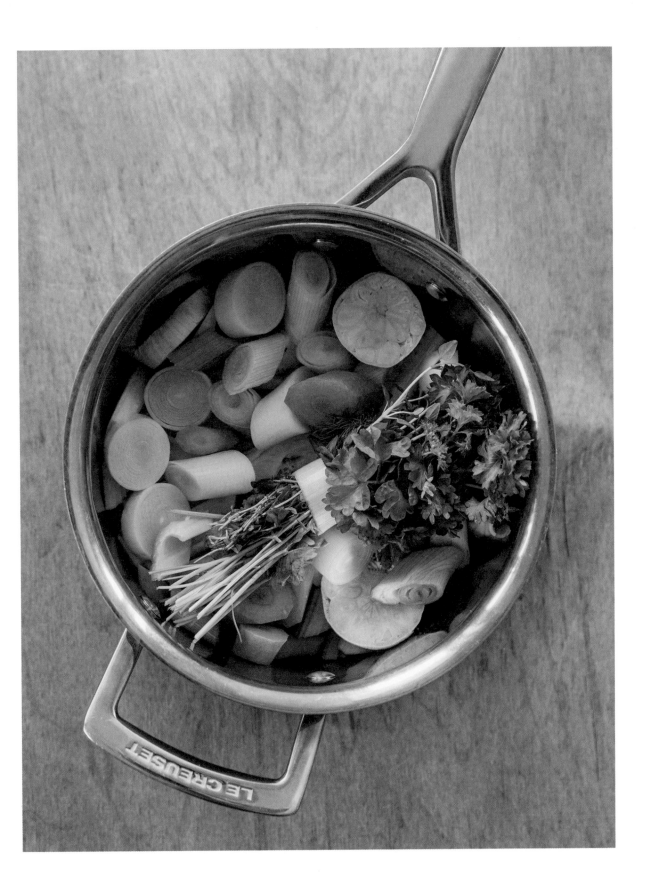

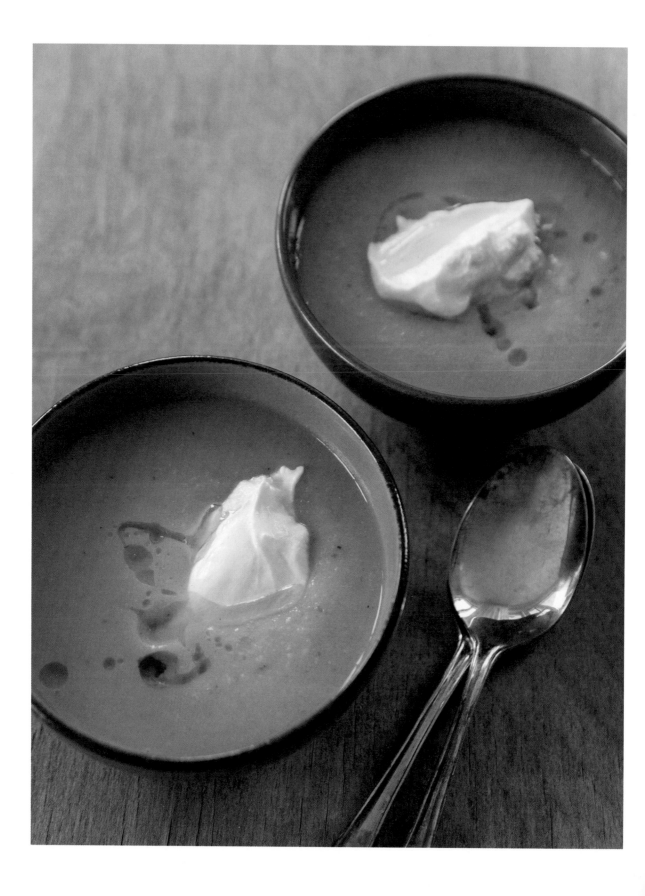

Coconut oil causes debate among nutritionists: avoid as high in saturated fat or eat as part of a balanced diet as it increases good cholesterol and encourages weight loss? There's no simple answer – I use it in my cooking, but generally when it makes sense for flavour. This recipe is a good example: why use anything else to make a curried coconut soup?

The benefits of carrots and sweet potatoes are less controversial: both are a good source of dietary fibre and they are also packed with beta-carotene, which really does help you see in the dark – useful when your headtorch batteries run out! Roasting them gives the soup a much deeper flavour, but if you are tight on time, just add them to the saucepan after sweating the onions and spices.

ROASTED CARROT, SWEET POTATO AND COCONUT SOUP WITH SPICED COCONUT OIL

SERVES 4-6

500g (1¼lb) carrots, coarsely chopped
500g (1¼lb) sweet potatoes, coarsely chopped
5 tbsp coconut oil
2 tsp curry powder (as hot as you like)
1 tsp ground turmeric
1 tsp coriander seeds
½ tsp cumin seeds
½ tsp dried chilli flakes (optional, plus extra to taste)
1 tsp sea salt
3 garlic cloves, crushed
1 large yellow onion, coarsely chopped
1 x 400ml (1²/₃ cups) can coconut milk
full-fat Greek or Turkish yogurt, to serve
fresh coriander (cilantro) leaves, to serve (optional)

1. Preheat the oven to 180°C/350°F/Gas 4.

2. Put the carrots and potatoes into a roasting pan and toss with 2 tablespoons coconut oil to coat. Roast for 45 minutes until softened and slightly golden.

3. Coarsely grind the spices together with the salt in a pestle and mortar.

4. Heat 1 tablespoon coconut oil in a large heavy saucepan over a medium heat, add the garlic and most of the spice mixture, reserving 1 teaspoon. Cook, stirring, for 1 minute, until the garlic is lightly golden. Add the onion, reduce the heat to low and cook for 5 minutes until the onion is starting to soften. Add the carrots, potatoes and enough water to cover and bring to the boil. Add the coconut milk, reduce the heat and simmer for 20 minutes.

5. Meanwhile, heat 2 tablespoons coconut oil in a small saucepan over a low heat, add the reserved spice mix and cook for 5 minutes. Strain the spiced oil through a fine sieve, discarding the spices, and set the oil aside.

6. With a hand-held stick blender or blender, purée the soup as you prefer (I like it with a little texture). Divide among serving bowls, top each with a spoonful of yogurt and drizzle over the spiced oil. You can add fresh coriander leaves or extra chilli flakes at this point, to taste.

A classic autumnal Tuscan peasant dish, this gives you the sustenance you would need for a long day out in the fields. It's not the most glamourous of dishes, but it's hard to beat when the leaves are turning and there's a bit of a chill in the air. It's a great recovery dish, as the beans are high in protein and the kale is packed with iron.

TUSCAN BEAN SOUP

SERVES 4

4 tbsp extra-virgin olive oil

2 carrots, coarsely diced

1 large onion, coarsely diced

3 celery stalks, coarsely diced

2 garlic cloves, crushed

3 thyme sprigs, leaves picked
  and chopped

1 litre (4 cups) chicken or vegetable
  stock

2 x 400g (14oz) cans white beans
  (cannellini are ideal)

250g (9oz) cavolo nero, stems
  removed, leaves finely chopped

salt and freshly ground black pepper,
  to taste

toast rubbed with raw garlic, and
  grated Parmesan cheese, to serve
  (optional)

1. Heat the olive oil in a large heavy saucepan over a low heat, add the carrots, onion, celery, garlic, thyme and ½ teaspoon salt and sweat the vegetables for 15–20 minutes until they are very soft but not coloured. Add the stock and beans and bring to the boil, then reduce the heat and simmer for 5 minutes. Add the cavolo nero and simmer for a further 5 minutes. Season with pepper and perhaps a little more salt.

2. This is lovely served in soup bowls with toast that has been rubbed with raw garlic and sprinkled with a little grated Parmesan cheese.

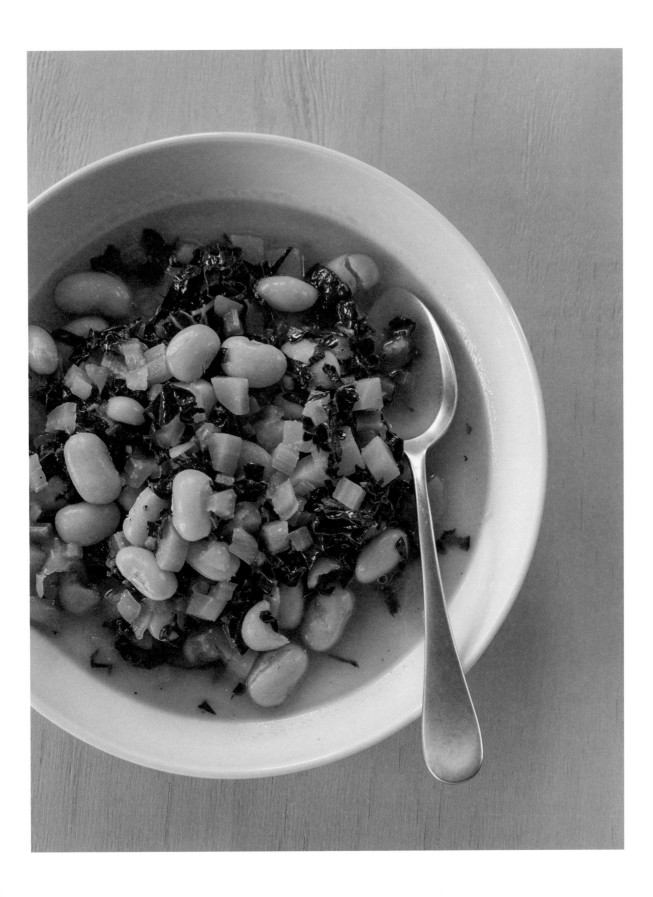

It's fun to challenge the way we think from time to time: in vegan circles, there's now a theory that molluscs are a less sophisticated organism than many plants, meaning they could be an excellent source of vegan protein. Molluscs are also high in vitamin B12 and omega 3, and low in fat. You can swap out the mussels for equally delicious clams here, too.

MUSSEL CHOWDER

SERVES 4

1kg (2¼lb) mussels

100ml (scant ½ cup) white wine

1 tbsp butter

2 white onions, finely diced

2 garlic cloves, crushed

400g (14oz) potatoes, peeled and chopped into 2cm (¾in) pieces

200g (7oz) sweetcorn kernels (ideally fresh from the cob but you can use frozen)

900ml (3¾ cups) vegetable stock (or use the recipe on p.70)

100ml (scant ½ cup) double or whipping cream (optional)

a handful of chopped flat-leaf parsley

salt and freshly ground black pepper, to taste

1. Pick through the mussels, removing the beards and discarding any with cracked shells or that remain open if you gently try to close them. Rinse under cold running water, then allow to drain in a colander for a couple of minutes.

2. Heat a large saucepan with a lid over a high heat until really hot, then add the mussels and wine, cover and cook for about 5 minutes until all the mussels have opened. Strain in a colander set over a bowl, reserving the cooking liquor. Allow to cool.

3. In the same saucepan, heat the butter over a low heat, add the onions and garlic and sweat for 10 minutes until translucent and softened. Add the potatoes and sweetcorn and gently cook for a further 2 minutes. Pour in the mussel liquor through a fine sieve and add the vegetable stock. Bring up to a low simmer and cook for about 10 minutes until the potato is cooked through.

4. Meanwhile, pick the mussel meat from the shells, discarding any that remained closed. Add the mussels to the finished chowder, taste and season with salt and plenty of black pepper. (I don't think it's necessary, but if you feel like treating yourself, add the cream at this point.) Bring up to a simmer, then remove from the heat.

5. Divide the mussel chowder among 4 soup bowls and top each with a large pinch of chopped parsley.

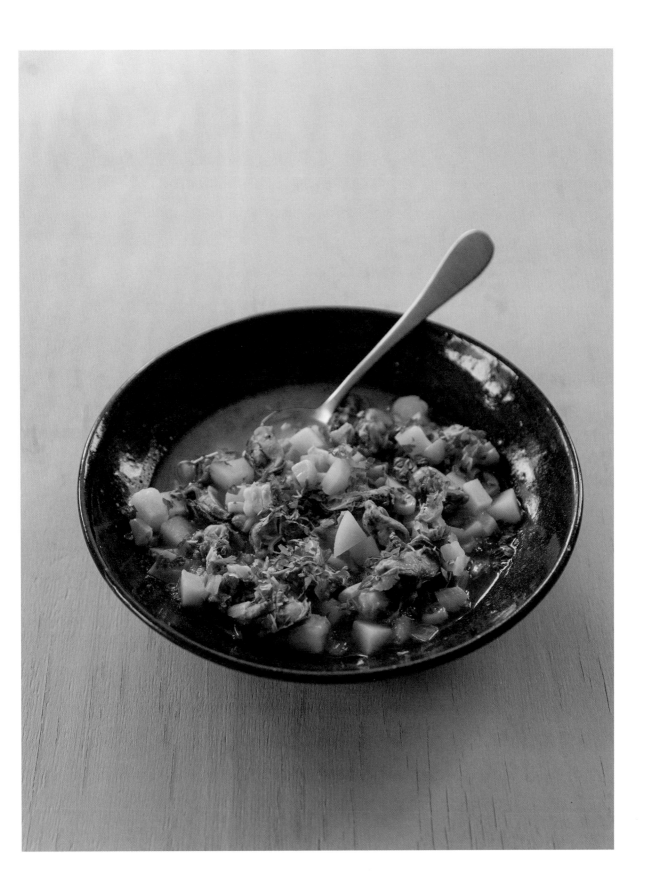

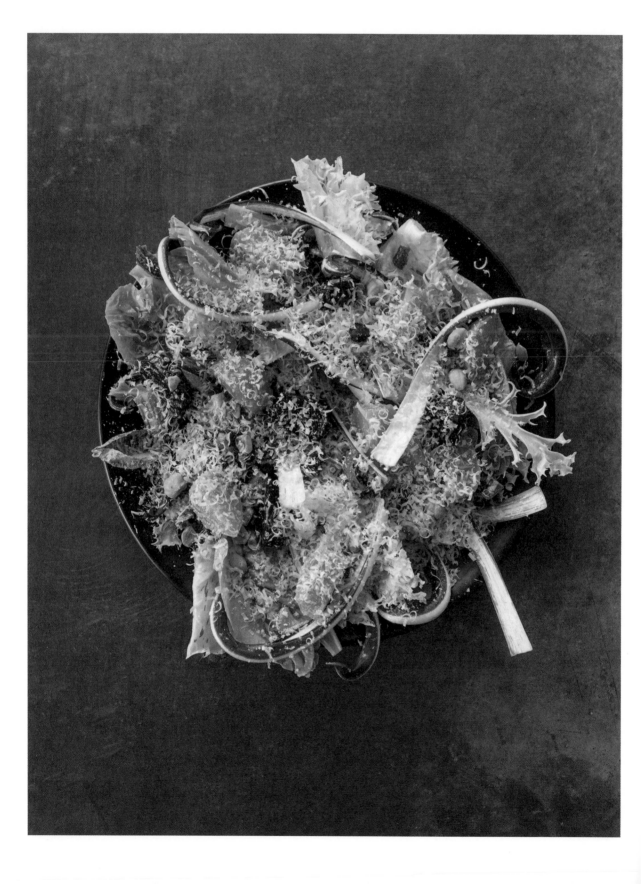

Salads

This salad is so beautiful. The bitter leaves can take getting used to, but balanced as they are with the sweet beetroot and salty, creamy cheese, it's a great way to get used to them! The chopped dates bring a welcome burst of sweetness to every other bite. Chicory and radicchio are known as prebiotics, meaning they promote good bacteria in the gut, as well as being packed with a whole host of other micronutrients.

WINTER BEETROOT SALAD

SERVES 4

800g (1¾lb) mixed beetroot (red and yellow)

a handful of hazelnuts

4 tbsp extra-virgin olive oil, plus extra for roasting

800g (1¾lb) mixed bitter Italian salad leaves (such as radicchio, endive/chicory, trevisano, castelfranco or tardivo), washed and pulled apart

2 tbsp red wine vinegar

8 pitted dates, chopped

150g (5oz) Pecorino cheese

sea salt, to taste

1. Boil the beetroot in a saucepan of boiling water until tender, about 30 minutes. Drain and allow to cool slightly, then peel and cut into wedges.

2. Preheat the oven to 180°C/350°F/Gas 4.

3. Spread the hazelnuts on a baking tray and toast in the oven for 8 minutes. Remove and allow to cool slightly, then coarsely chop and set aside.

4. Transfer the beetroot to a large bowl and mix with a glug of olive oil and a pinch of salt. Spread the wedges over a baking tray and roast for 20 minutes. Keep warm until ready to serve.

5. In a large mixing bowl, lightly toss the bitter salad leaves with the 4 tablespoons of olive oil, red wine vinegar and a pinch of salt. Taste and add more salt or vinegar if you feel the need.

6. Divide the leaves among 4 large shallow bowls. Top each serving with roasted beets and evenly scatter over the hazelnuts and chopped dates. Use a fine grater or microplane to grate the Pecorino cheese over each salad. Serve immediately.

I think this salad is hard to beat after a hot summer run. Watermelon is great for rehydration, and full of natural sugars and vitamin C. The asparagus is high in fibre and, as a prebiotic, it encourages healthy gut bacteria. The slight bitterness of the asparagus and saltiness of the feta balance out the sweetness of the watermelon very nicely.

WATERMELON, CHARRED ASPARAGUS AND FETA SALAD

SERVES 4

1 cucumber, sliced lengthways

2 bunches of asparagus, woody parts removed, halved

4 tbsp extra-virgin olive oil

2 tbsp white wine vinegar

½ medium watermelon, peeled and chopped into 2cm (¾in) pieces

200g (7oz) feta cheese, crumbled

1 small red onion, sliced into thin rings and rinsed for 1 minute in cold water

a bunch of basil leaves, picked

dried Turkish chilli flakes, to taste (optional)

sea salt, to taste

1. Heat a dry cast-iron frying pan over a high heat until smoking hot, then put the cucumber in, flesh-side down, and cook for 3–4 minutes until the flesh is charred. Remove from the pan, cut into uneven bite-size chunks and set aside in a large bowl.

2. Add the asparagus to the same pan and cook, stirring, for 4–5 minutes until the asparagus has softened slightly and is evenly charred.

3. Mix the asparagus with the cucumber in the bowl, along with the olive oil, white wine vinegar and a pinch of salt. Add the watermelon, then check that you are happy with the seasoning.

4. Divide the salad among 4 salad bowls, then top with the crumbled feta, onion rings, basil leaves and chilli flakes (if using).

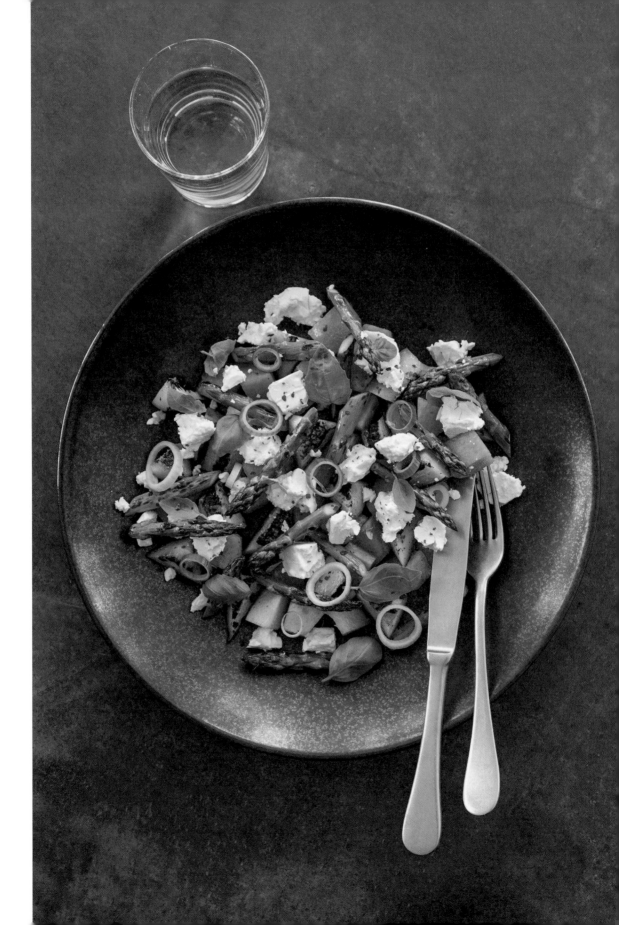

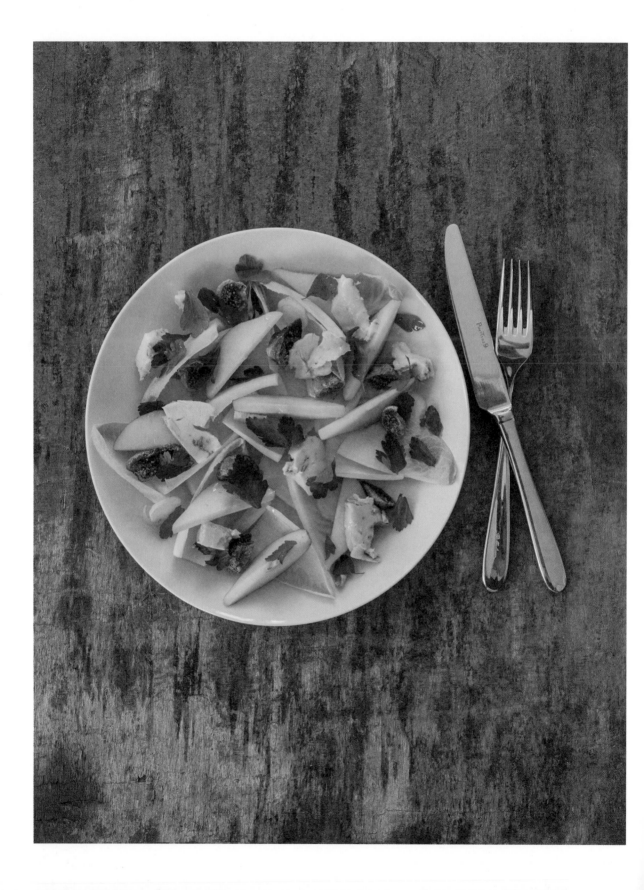

This is a play on the classic 1970s Waldorf salad. The endive (chicory) is a prebiotic and Gorgonzola a probiotic, so both help promote healthy and diverse bacteria in the stomach. The pear and dried fig bring sweetness to balance the bitterness of the endive and salt from the cheese, while also adding some slow-burning sugars as a source of energy. Remember to remove the cheese from the refrigerator 30 minutes before you plan to eat this, to allow it to get to room temperature.

ENDIVE AND GORGONZOLA SALAD

SERVES 4

4 heads of white endive (chicory), leaves separated and halved

1 tbsp white wine vinegar

2 tbsp extra-virgin olive oil, plus extra for drizzling

a pinch of sea salt

6 small dried figs, quartered

4 small ripe pears, cored and sliced (Williams or Conference are my favourites)

200g (7oz) Gorgonzola, at room temperature

a handful of flat-leaf parsley, leaves picked and very coarsely chopped

1. In a mixing bowl, dress the endive leaves with the white wine vinegar, olive oil and the salt.

2. Divide the leaves between 4 shallow bowls or plates, then top each with dried figs and slices of pear. Spoon several blobs of Gorgonzola onto each serving and finish with the chopped parsley and an extra drizzle of olive oil.

This salad is commonplace in Turkey, although I first saw it in Diana Henry's wonderful book, *Simple*. Chickpeas, and in fact all pulses, are a good source of vegetarian protein, the cauliflower is high in fibre, and the pomegranate is packed with vitamin C and all sorts of antioxidants.

ROAST CAULIFLOWER, CHICKPEA, OLIVE AND POMEGRANATE SALAD WITH HUMMUS

SERVES 4

2 x cauliflower heads, separated into quite small florets

3 tbsp extra-virgin olive oil, plus extra for drizzling

1 x 400g (14oz) can chickpeas, drained and rinsed

1 x 200g (7oz) jar Kalamata olives, drained (I like them with the stone left in, but it's up to you)

juice of ½ lemon

seeds of 1 pomegranate

a large handful of flat-leaf parsley leaves

sea salt and freshly ground black pepper, to taste

FOR THE HUMMUS:

1 x 200g (7oz) can chickpeas, drained and rinsed

2 tbsp tahini

1 tsp crushed roasted cumin seeds

1 small garlic clove, crushed with a little salt

4-5 tbsp extra-virgin olive oil

a squeeze of lemon juice

sea salt, to taste

1. Preheat the oven to 220°C/425°F/Gas 7.

2. Put the cauliflower florets into a roasting pan, drizzle with 2 tablespoons olive oil and season with a pinch of salt. Roast for 10–15 minutes until golden brown, stirring once or twice so that they colour evenly.

3. Meanwhile, make the hummus. Pulse the chickpeas, tahini, cumin and garlic in a food processor until slightly broken down. Add the olive oil and process until smooth (you may need to add a little extra olive oil). Season with a pinch of salt and a squeeze of lemon juice, then taste to see if you need to add more salt, lemon or garlic. If you are planning on running later in the day, be careful how much garlic you go for! Set aside.

4. Remove the cauliflower from the oven and transfer to a salad bowl. Mix in the chickpeas and olives, then dress with the remaining 1 tablespoon olive oil and the lemon juice. Season with a pinch of salt and a few grindings of black pepper. Leave the ingredients to get to know one another for 5 minutes or so, before gently mixing in the pomegrate seeds.

5. To serve, spread the hummus over 4 plates. Pile the cauliflower salad on top of the hummus, top generously with the parsley and finish with a drizzle of olive oil.

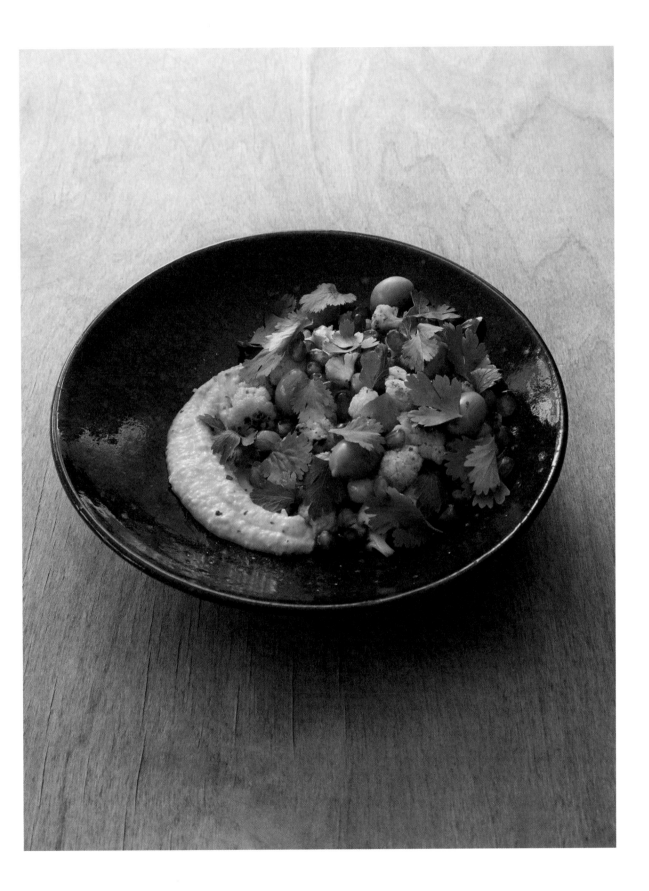

I love squid – simply pan-fried or grilled with a fresh salad, it is impossible to beat. Squid is a really good source of protein and, although it may look at little intimidating, is easy to cook. If you ask nicely, your local fishmonger or supermarket fish counter will clean and score the squid for you.

SQUID, TOMATO AND AVOCADO SALAD WITH LIME AND CORIANDER

SERVES 4

2 medium squid, cleaned and scored

extra-virgin olive oil, for drizzling

1 small red onion, finely diced

2–3 limes: 1 juiced (or more to taste); 1–2 cut into halves or wedges to serve

1kg (2¼lb) ripe mixed tomatoes (ideally on the vine), chopped into bite-size chunks

1 small romaine lettuce, coarsely chopped

a bunch of fresh coriander (cilantro), chopped

2 ripe avocados, flesh only, cut into bite-size chunks

coarse sea salt, to taste

a pinch of chilli flakes (optional), to serve

1. Combine the squid in a large bowl with a drizzle of olive oil and a pinch of salt and set aside to marinate for about 5 minutes.

2. Combine the red onion in a mixing bowl with a pinch of salt and the lime juice. Leave the ingredients to get to know one another for 10 minutes.

3. Add the tomatoes, lettuce and fresh coriander to the onion mixture.

4. Heat a cast-iron frying pan over a high heat until smoking hot, then add the marinated squid to the pan (you may want to do this in 2 batches, so as not to cool the pan down too much). Sear for 1 minute on each side until the body flesh has curled up and the tentacles have a little golden colour, then remove from the pan.

5. Chop the squid into bite-size pieces and add to the salad.

6. Finally, add the avocado to the salad, along with a glug of olive oil, then taste to see whether you need to add more salt or lime juice. Arrange in 4 shallow bowls and serve sprinkled with chilli flakes (if using), with lime halves or wedges on the side and – who could forget – some ice-cold beer.

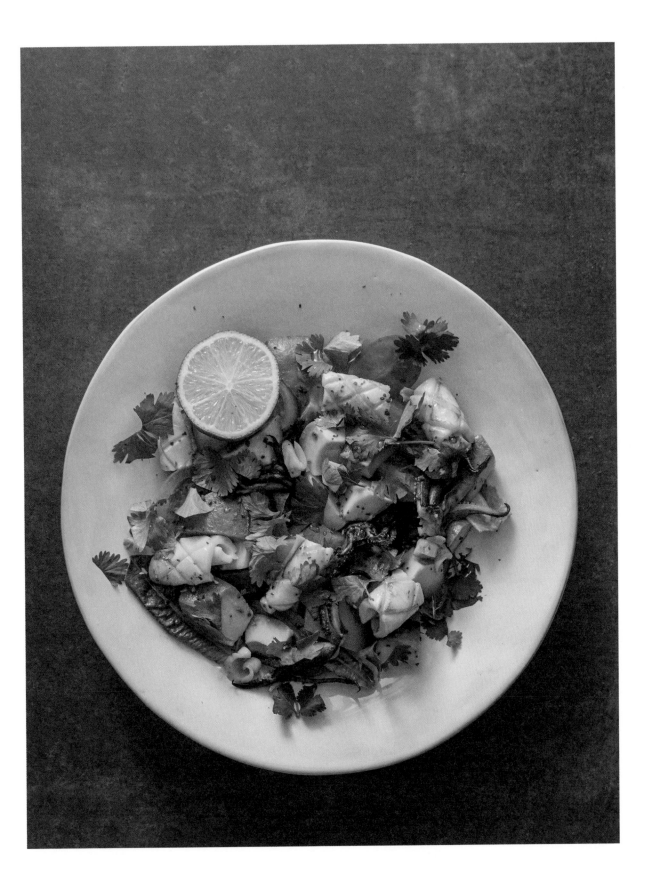

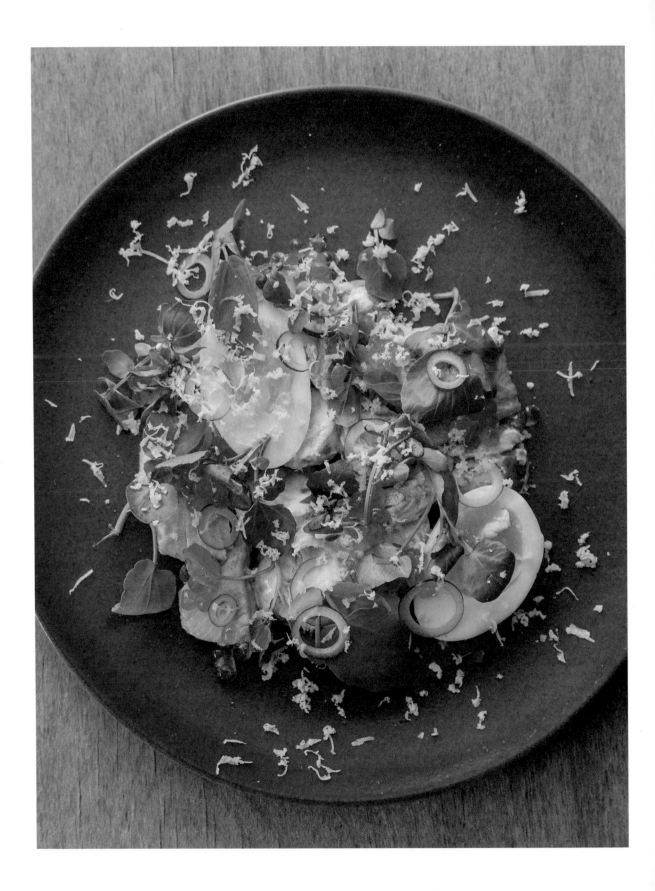

Rainbow trout is an excellent source of protein and is high in omega 3 fatty acids, which are essential for a healthy heart. Interestingly, cold or room-temperature boiled potatoes are higher in dietary fibre and a slower burning carbohydrate than when eaten warm – strange, but true. The horseradish gives this a great kick and I love the salty little bursts of trout roe.

RAINBOW TROUT, POTATO AND EGG SALAD WITH HORSERADISH DRESSING

SERVES 4

400g (14oz) new potatoes

4 eggs

100g (3¾oz) sour cream

2 tbsp extra-virgin olive oil, plus extra for drizzling

1 tsp Dijon mustard

juice of ½ lemon

about 50g (2oz) fresh horseradish, peeled

100g (3¾oz) watercress, loosely picked

400g (14oz) steamed rainbow trout

1 small red onion, sliced into rings, rinsed in cold water for 1 minute

50g (2oz) trout roe (optional)

sea salt, to taste

1. Boil the new potatoes in a saucepan of lightly salted water until just tender, about 10 minutes. Drain and set aside.

2. Meanwhile, boil the eggs for 6 minutes in a separate saucepan of water. Drain and cool under running water, then peel and halve.

3. In a small bowl, combine the sour cream, olive oil, mustard and lemon juice. Use a fine grater or microplane to grate in the horseradish, reserving some for the garnish (I like it really strong, but you can put in as much as you feel comfortable with). Add a pinch of salt, then gently mix in the potatoes, trying to avoid breaking them up too much.

4. Divide the dressed potatoes among 4 salad bowls or plates or spread over a large serving dish. Top with the watercress and gently flake over the trout. Top with the egg halves, red onion rings and a few dots of trout roe (if using), then finish with a drizzle of olive oil and the reserved grated horseradish.

I love this! The salmon is fatty enough to handle the robust flavours of soy and sesame and the cucumber salad is amazing. Salmon is a good source of protein and full of omega 3 fatty acids. I briefly freeze fish that I'm going to serve raw or cured, to ensure any parasites have been killed off. Always use wild or farmed salmon with the MSC mark, to be sure it has been sustainably sourced.

CURED SALMON WITH SMASHED CUCUMBER AND AVOCADO MAYONNAISE

SERVES 4

FOR THE CURED SALMON:

400g (14oz) fresh salmon fillet, skinned (defrosted if previously frozen)

5 tbsp soy sauce

2 tbsp sesame oil

1 tsp sugar (any type)

FOR THE SMASHED CUCUMBER:

2 cucumbers

1 garlic clove, crushed

2 tbsp soy sauce

1 tbsp sesame oil

2 tsp rice wine vinegar

½ tsp dried chilli flakes

½ tsp sugar (any type)

½ tsp fish sauce

FOR THE AVOCADO MAYONNAISE:

2 ripe avocados, flesh only, coarsely chopped

1 tsp Dijon mustard

juice of ½ lime, or more to taste

a pinch of sea salt, or more to taste

50ml (¼ cup) mild extra-virgin olive oil

TO SERVE:

1 tbsp sesame seeds

a handful of fresh coriander (cilantro) leaves

1. Ideally the day before but at least 6 hours before you plan to eat, place the salmon in a zip-lock bag. Mix together the soy sauce, sesame oil and sugar, pour over the salmon to cover, then seal and place in the refrigerator.

2. When ready to serve, remove the cured fish from the refrigerator 30 minutes beforehand, to bring it to room temperature.

3. To make the smashed cucumber, use a rolling pin to bash the cucumbers a few times, just firmly enough to soften and break down the insides a bit. Cut the bruised cucumbers in half lengthways, then into 1cm (²⁄₅in) slices. Place in a mixing bowl, add the remaining ingredients, mix well and allow to marinate for at least 15 minutes.

4. To make the mayonnaise, combine the avocado, mustard, lime juice and salt in a bowl. Use a hand-held stick blender to blend to a paste. With the blender still running, slowly drizzle in the oil, blending until the mixture forms a thick mayo. Taste and add more salt or lime juice if necessary.

5. Drain the salmon of its marinade and cut it into slices, about 5mm (¹⁄₅in) thick. Arrange on serving plates with a pile of the smashed cucumber salad and a little of its marinade, then add a spoonful of the mayonnaise. Serve, sprinkled with sesame seeds and fresh coriander.

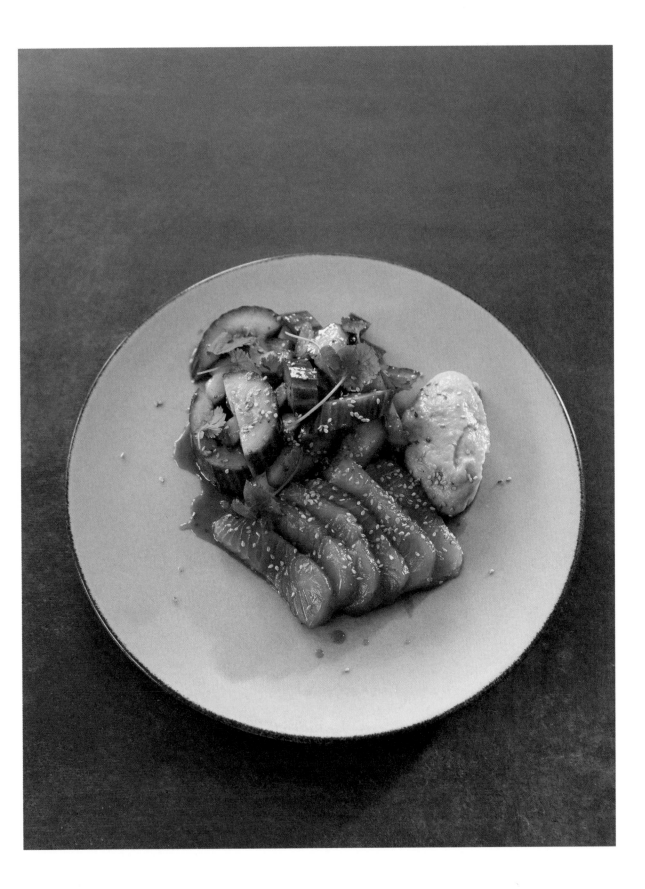

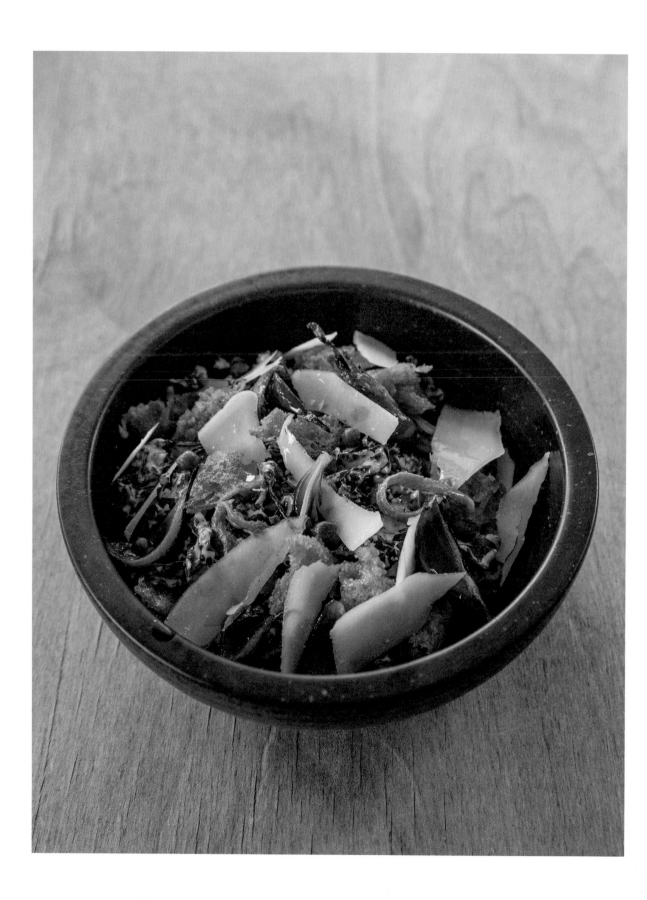

I love Caesar salad, but unfortunately it's rare to get a really good one. I swapped the usual cos lettuce for cavolo nero in this recipe, since it gives a deep savoury flavour and stands up to the rather aggressive garlic and anchovies in the dressing. This recipe makes probably twice the amount of dressing you'll need, but it's hard to make lesser quantities and it keeps well in a covered container in the refrigerator for up to a week.

CAVOLO NERO CAESAR SALAD

SERVES 4

3 red onions, cut into wedges

olive oil, for drizzling

⅓ loaf of day-old bread, crusts removed (to give about 200g /7oz), torn into pieces

800g (1¾lb) cavolo nero, stalks removed, coarsely chopped

8 anchovy fillets

2 tsp capers

100g (3¾oz) Parmesan cheese, shaved with a peeler

sea salt and freshly ground black pepper, to taste

FOR THE DRESSING:

1 garlic clove, crushed

1 egg yolk

3 anchovy fillets

1 tsp Dijon mustard

100g (3¾oz) Parmesan cheese, finely grated

200ml (scant 1 cup) olive oil

2 tbsp sour cream

sea salt and freshly ground black pepper, to taste

1. Preheat the oven to 180°C/350°F/Gas 4.

2. Coat the red onion wedges with a drizzle of olive oil and a pinch of salt and place in a roasting pan. Roast for 20 minutes.

3. Meanwhile, coat the bread pieces with some more olive oil and plenty of black pepper. Add to the onions in the roasting pan for the final 7–8 minutes of cooking time and roast until golden brown. Both the onions and croutons should be ready at the same time and the bread will have soaked up some of the onion roasting juices.

4. To make the dressing, combine the garlic, egg yolk, anchovy fillets, mustard and Parmesan in a bowl, and blend with a hand-held stick blender or whisk together by hand. With the blender still running, or while continuing to whisk, slowly pour in the olive oil, mixing until the dressing comes together like a mayonnaise. When all the olive oil is incorporated, add the sour cream and gently fold it in with a spoon.

5. In a large bowl, mix the cavolo nero with half the dressing, half the roasted red onion and half the croutons until everything is well coated. Taste and season with more salt or pepper, if needed (remember the capers and anchovies are salty).

6. Divide among 4 bowls and top with the remaining red onions and croutons. Tear the anchovy fillets into strips and place a couple of pieces on each serving, then add a few capers and Parmesan shavings to finish.

Pizza

'Real' food is something that all the runners I know try to eat at some point during a race. I know from my own experience that having something to look forward to, even something as mundane as a slice of cold pizza, can give the spirits a boost during the darker moments of a long race.

If I'm at home the evening before a race, I'll generally bake pizza, adding plenty of seeds and whole grains to the dough. It's a good dinner that the whole family enjoys and I find easily digestible. Then, if the race the following day is longer than about 30 miles (50km), I put leftover slices into freezer bags and add them to my racepack or to a dropbag, if there is one.

If you have a baking stone, these are perfect to use for baking pizzas, otherwise a really hot baking tray lined with baking paper will do the trick.

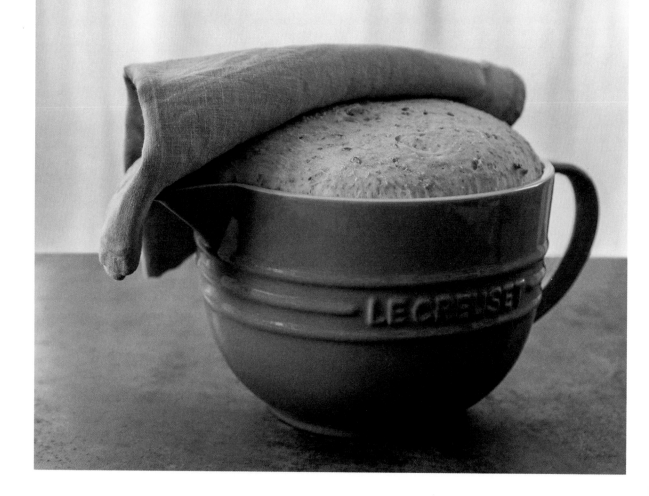

BASIC PIZZA DOUGH

500g (1¼b) strong white bread flour, plus extra for dusting

100g (3¾oz) wholewheat flour

1½ tbsp chia seeds

2 tbsp flax seeds (linseeds)

2 tsp (10g /²/₅oz) active dried yeast

450ml (scant 2 cups) warm water

1 cup (280g/2dl) Sourdough Starter (see p.183)

2 tsp (10g/²/₅oz) salt

1. Combine the flours, chia and flax seeds in a large bowl or in a stand mixer.

2. In a separate bowl or jug, mix the yeast with the warm water and starter.

3. Slowly add the yeast mixture to the flour mixture and mix with your hands or in the machine until you have a rather wet dough. Cover with a clean tea towel and allow to rest for 10 minutes.

4. Add the salt to the dough, mixing until incorporated, then knead for 10 minutes until it becomes firmer and feels more elastic and strong. Place back in the bowl, cover with the tea towel and allow to rest in a warm place for 1 hour until almost doubled in size. Alternatively, make it the day before and refrigerate overnight for a more sour-flavoured dough.

5. Scoop the dough onto the work surface, divide into 6 equal pieces and shape each into a rough ball. Cover with a clean tea towel and allow to rise for 30 minutes until plump in appearance.

6. Meanwhile, preheat the oven to 250°C/500°F/Gas 10 or to as hot as it goes. Place your baking stone (or a baking tray lined with baking paper) in the oven to heat up.

7. On a work surface dusted with a little flour, flatten one of the dough balls with your hand to a disc about 1cm (²/₅in) thick, then use a rolling pin to roll it out to about 25cm (10in) in diameter. You may need to keep dusting the work surface, so the dough doesn't stick. Transfer the pizza base to a thin chopping board dusted with flour (this way, you can transfer the pizza to the oven with minimal risk of dropping it on the floor).

8. Add your toppings (see Pizza Toppings, pp.96–97).

9. Bake each pizza base, ideally one by one, for 5–7 minutes, or until the toppings are golden brown and the base is coloured and slightly charred in places.

Pizza Toppings

Top the pizzas with whatever you feel like. These are a few of my go-to recipes. If you plan to use leftovers for race nutrition the following day, remember not to use toppings that may be difficult to digest on the move. Anchovies or spicy pepperoni are not good options, in my experience.

Each recipe makes enough to top 1 pizza, apart from the tomato sauce, which should be enough to top 6 pizzas. If you have any leftover tomato sauce, it will keep for 2–3 days in an airtight container in the refrigerator or could be added to a tomato sauce for pasta.

GOATS' CHEESE, BEETROOT AND POTATO

4–5 cooked new potatoes
extra-virgin olive oil, for drizzling
2 tbsp crème fraîche
2–3 cooked beetroot (mixed colours), peeled and thinly sliced
100g (3¾oz) goats' cheese, crumbled

1. In a bowl, crush the cooked new potatoes slightly and dress with olive oil.

2. Spoon the crème fraîche onto the pizza base, top with the crushed potatoes, beetroot slices and crumbled goats' cheese, then drizzle with a little more olive oil.

3. Bake the pizza according to instructions on p.95.

CAVOLO NERO, CHARD AND MOZZARELLA

4–5 cavolo nero leaves (or other kale), chopped
4–5 chard leaves, chopped
olive oil, for drizzling
2 tbsp crème fraîche
1 mozzarella ball, torn

1. In a bowl, dress the chopped cavolo nero and chard with a little olive oil.

2. Spoon the crème fraîche onto the pizza base, top with the dressed greens and scatter over the mozzarella. Drizzle with any leftover oil from the greens.

3. Bake the pizza according to instructions on p.95.

AUBERGINE, TOMATO AND MOZZARELLA

olive oil, for frying
1 aubergine (eggplant), thinly sliced
1 mozzarella ball, torn
1 tsp capers
a small handful of black olives

FOR THE TOMATO SAUCE:
1 x 400g (14oz) can good-quality chopped
   tomatoes
a generous glug of extra-virgin olive oil
a pinch of salt

1. To make the sauce, drain the tomatoes in a fine sieve for 1–2 minutes. Transfer the tomato pulp to a bowl and mix with a generous glug of olive oil and a pinch of salt.

2. Heat a glug of olive oil in a frying pan over a medium heat, add the aubergine and fry for about 2 minutes on each side until golden brown.

3. Spoon 2 tablespoons of the tomato sauce onto the pizza base and spread evenly. Top with a few fried aubergine slices and the mozzarella, then scatter over the capers and black olives.

4. Bake the pizza according to instructions on p.95.

TOMATO, CAPER, OLIVE AND PECORINO

2 fresh tomatoes, chopped
½ red onion, very thinly sliced
extra-virgin olive oil, for drizzling
a small handful of black olives
1 tbsp small capers
100g (3¾oz) Pecorino cheese

FOR THE TOMATO SAUCE:
1 x 400g (14oz) can good-quality chopped
   tomatoes
a generous glug of extra-virgin olive oil
a pinch of salt

1. To make the sauce, drain the tomatoes in a fine sieve for 1–2 minutes. Transfer the tomato pulp to a bowl and mix with a generous glug of olive oil and a pinch of salt.

2. In a separate bowl, dress the fresh tomatoes and onion with a little olive oil.

3. Spoon 2 tablespoons of the tomato sauce onto the pizza base and spread out evenly. Scatter over the dressed tomato and red onion mixture, along with the olives and capers, then grate over the Pecorino cheese.

4. Bake the pizza according to instructions on p.95.

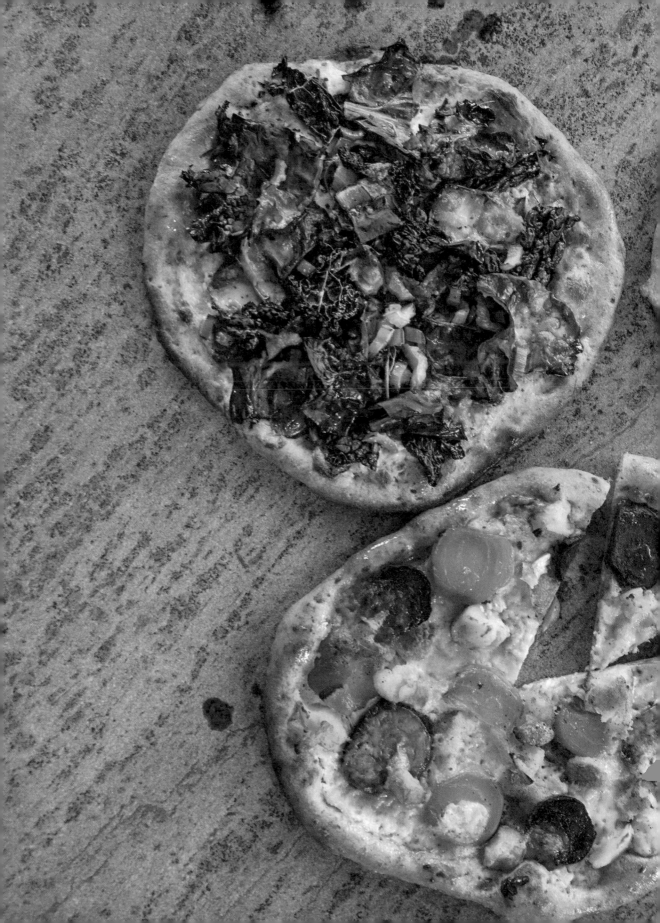

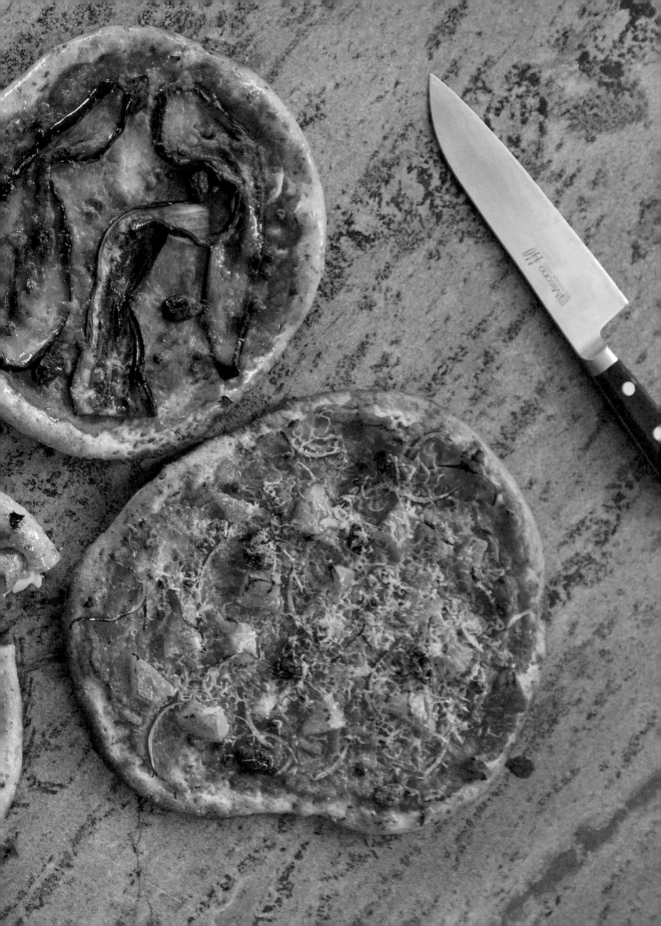

On the Trail with:

Ricky Lightfoot

The Lake District, UK

AS SOON AS THE EMBRYO of this book was formed, the very first place I thought to visit was the Lake District in the UK, where the dramatic ranges of hills and mountains (known locally as fells) take your breath away. It's the spiritual home of fell running – straight up, straight down, no frills or goodie bags, just real racing in the hills. In this small part of the world, the simple act of moving quickly across rugged land is still prized, and it's a place that I hold close to my heart.

I was to meet with Ricky Lightfoot, a Lakeland local and internationally acclaimed mountain runner. Inspired to get outside more by a love of the fells than by the glory that comes with being a top-level mountain runner, Ricky is the perfect

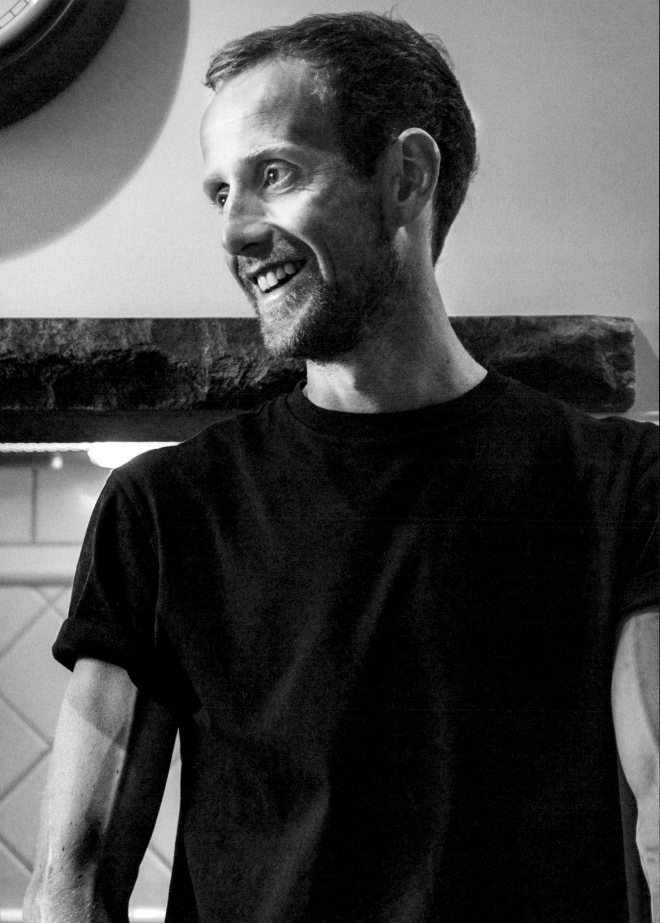

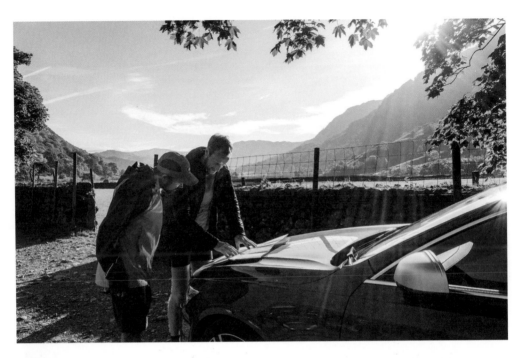

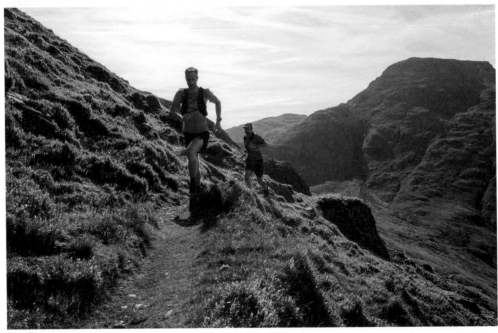

RICKY LIGHTFOOT

«It's more efficient for me to include a little carbohydrate in every meal leading up to an event, rather than having one big bowl of pasta the night before. If I overeat the night before, the food might not be fully digested before I start running the next day.»

---

guide to this area. He knows it like the back of his hand and promises that we are in for a treat.

On my drive down to the Lakes, the weather was exceptional and, with a few miles to go, I got my first glimpse of the fells. Every time I visit the Lake District, I feel like a kid at Christmas – I just want to pull the car over and get out and run up the nearest hill! I have spent a lot of time there and never been as fortunate to catch a couple of days as glorious as these. The views were breath-taking. I met Ricky at his house the evening before the Blencathra Fell Race, so (as is wise, pre-race) spicy food was off the menu that night. When it comes to food, Ricky allows himself to eat pretty much everything, not so much meat but certainly plenty of vegetables and fish. With this in mind, I decided to roast a spatchcocked chicken and serve it with quinoa tabbouleh and chicory (see p. 116). The tabbouleh was packed with herbs and vegetables and quinoa is a great source of unprocessed carbohydrates, so it was perfect for providing the energy we needed before a large effort.

Ricky's biggest self-confessed vice is cake (see p.153 for his outstanding Banana Bread recipe)! With weekly averages of 80–100 miles (129–160km) a week, he doesn't have to go without, but he does prefer to bake himself so that he knows exactly what is going into whatever he eats. Knowing this, I couldn't resist making him a honey, yogurt and olive oil cake (see p.159), with the best (and easiest) honey ice cream you can imagine (see p.159). His daughter, Isobelle, was especially looking forward to this part of the meal.

Ricky is a fireman in the small town of Workington, Cumbria, and has a young family, yet still manages to get out on the fells almost every day, ideally twice a day. Recalling his youth and starting out running, he says that he was far from the best among his running group, but his passion for the sport and clear love for getting out in the mountains has proven that, with hard work and determination, you can achieve great things. After a lovely evening spent listening to tales of the fells and about Ricky's life travelling as a runner, I left for an early night, ready for an early start in the morning.

We met at first light in the tiny village of Seathwaite in the West Lakes. Initially, we headed off up the steady incline to Scafell Pike, England's highest point, but bore to the right, up towards a less well-trodden part of the area. We traversed the scree fields of Little Hell Gate, scrambled up Arrowhead Ridge and to the top of Great Gable, with its awe-inspiring views across to Scafell Pike, down the Wasdale valley towards the Wastwater lake and on to the sea. It is such a beautiful and tranquil place; although we were out in the fells for almost four hours, we barely met a soul.

Arriving back at the car, we headed off in separate directions, arranging to meet later that

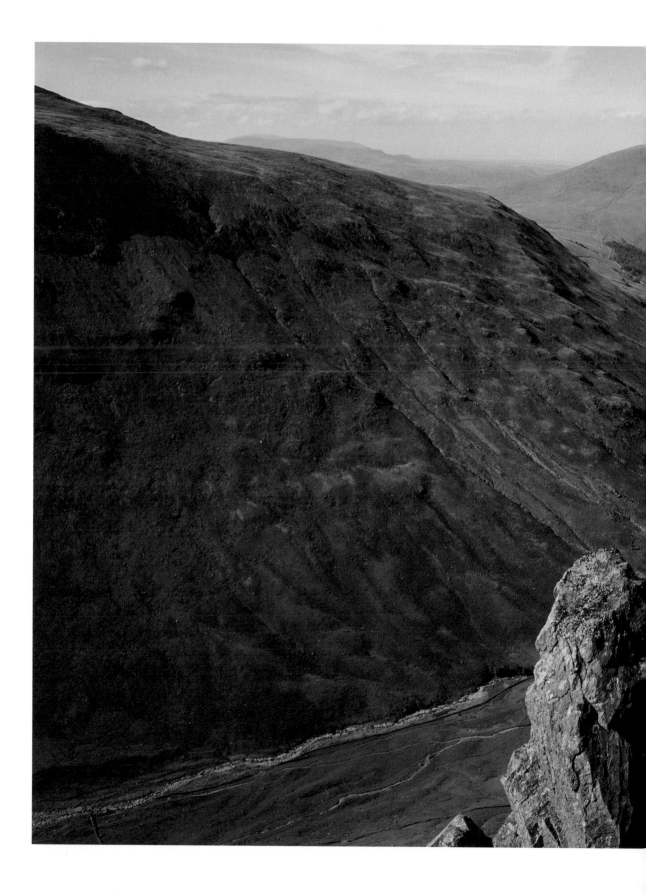

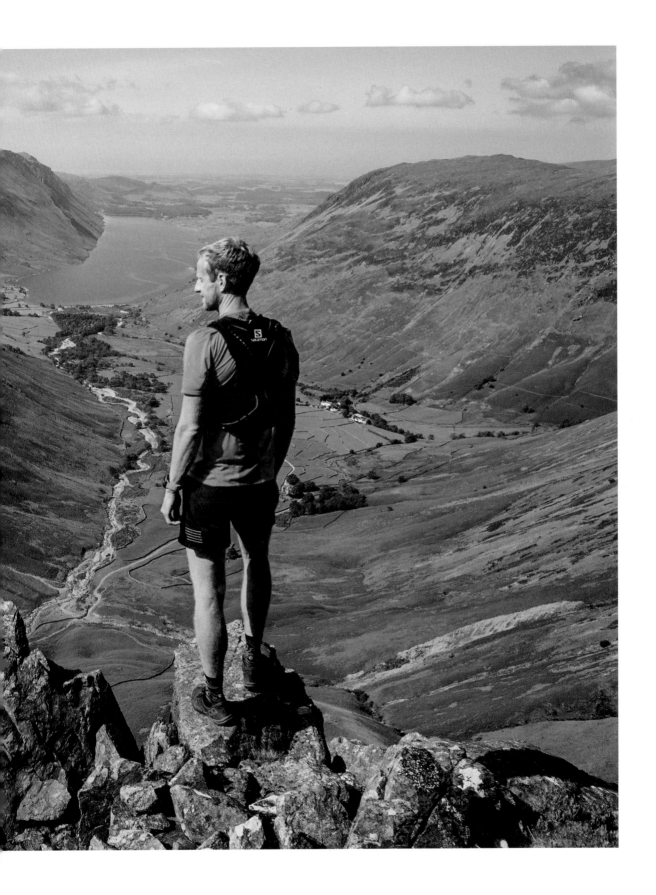

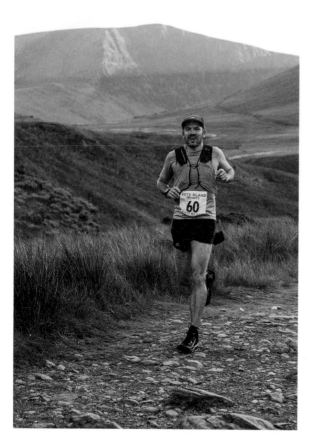

evening in Mungrisdale for the Blencathra Fell Race, a 7.6-mile (12km) loop up and down the fell to the summit of Blencathra, taking in 800 metres (2600 feet) of vertical gain. Ricky is the long-standing course record holder; with a blisteringly fast time of 58:29, he is one of only two people to have broken an hour on the course.

It was a beautiful evening and, with a turnout of well over a hundred people, it promised to be an exciting race! At seven o'clock prompt the starting pistol fired and off we went. Within the first 200 metres (650 feet) the route took us off trail and directly up the fell. In the distance, I could see Ricky already leading by some way, and that was the last I saw of him until I came panting to the finish line, one-and-a-half hours later. Ricky won the race in just over an hour, beating the second-placed runner by five minutes. I finished somewhere in the middle, exhausted but over the moon.

Fell running really is the purest form of running competition. There are no prizes, next to no entry fee, no sponsorship in sight, and it ends at the village pub with a well-deserved pint of local ale and a portion of chips. The perfect celebration of the sport. •

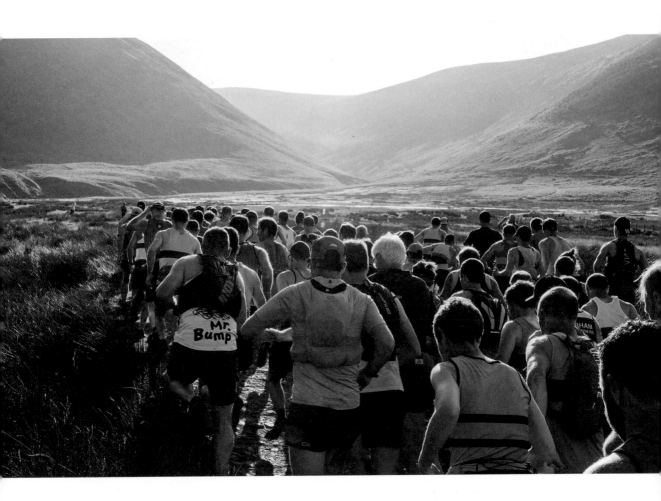

Race stats (selected)

Borrowdale Fell Race: six-times winner
2009 Blencathra Fell Race: win and course record
2009 Zegama-Aizkorri Marathon, Basque Country: winner
2013 World Trail Running Championships, Wales: winner
2013 Otter Trail, South Africa: win and course record (first non-South African winner)

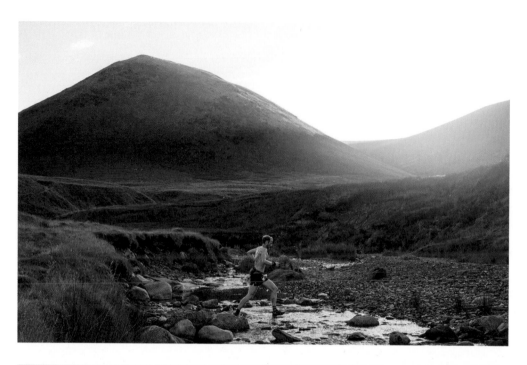

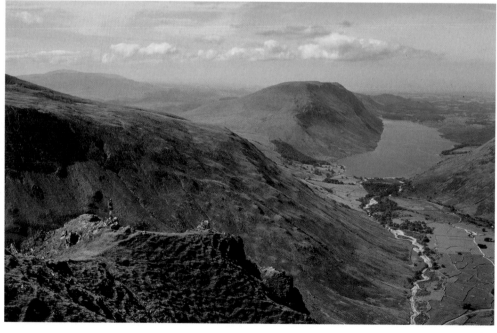

RICKY LIGHTFOOT

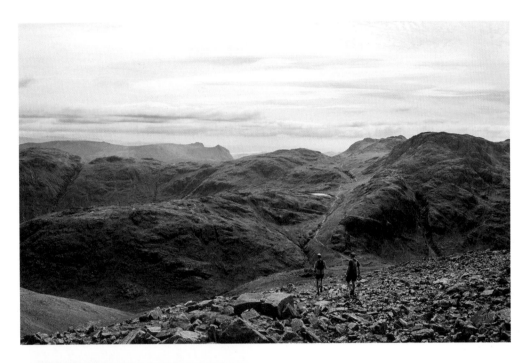

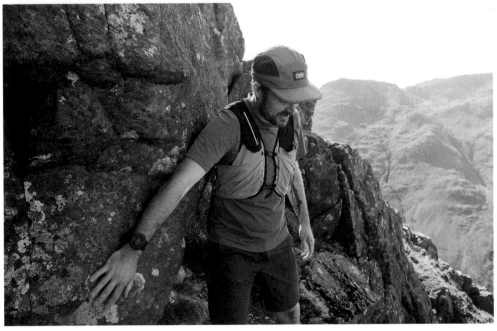

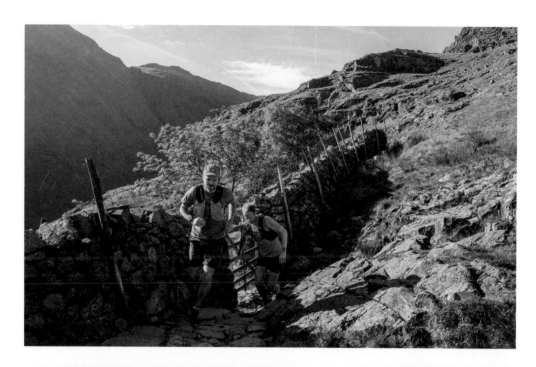

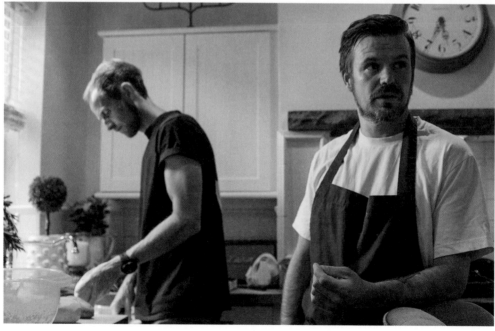

RICKY LIGHTFOOT

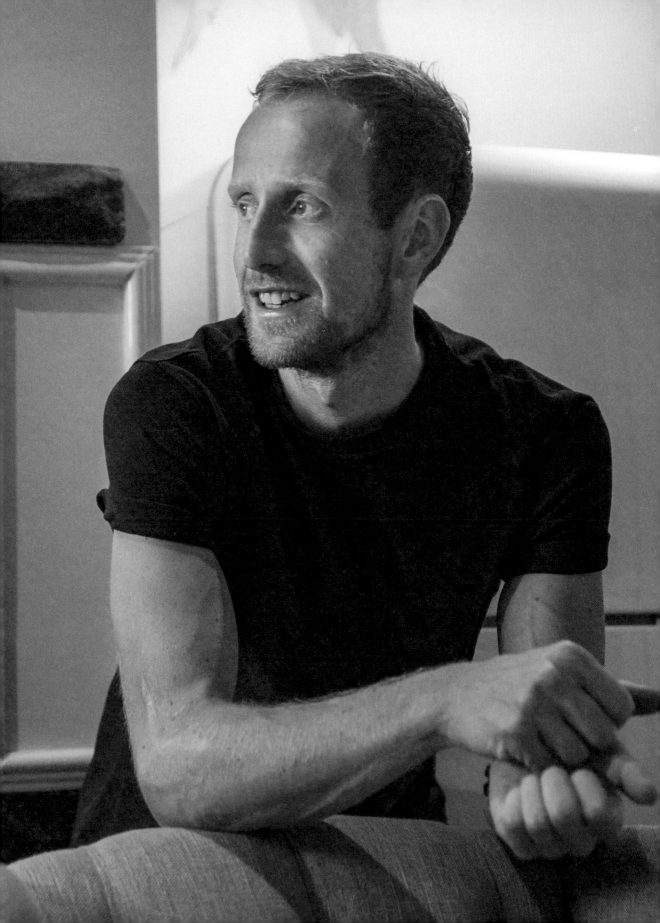

CHAPTER THREE

Dinner

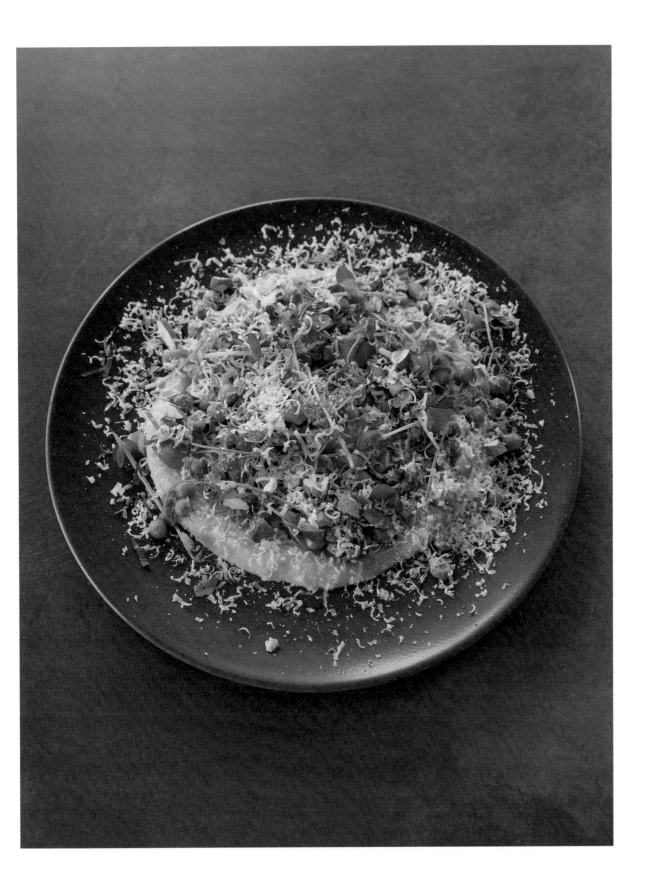

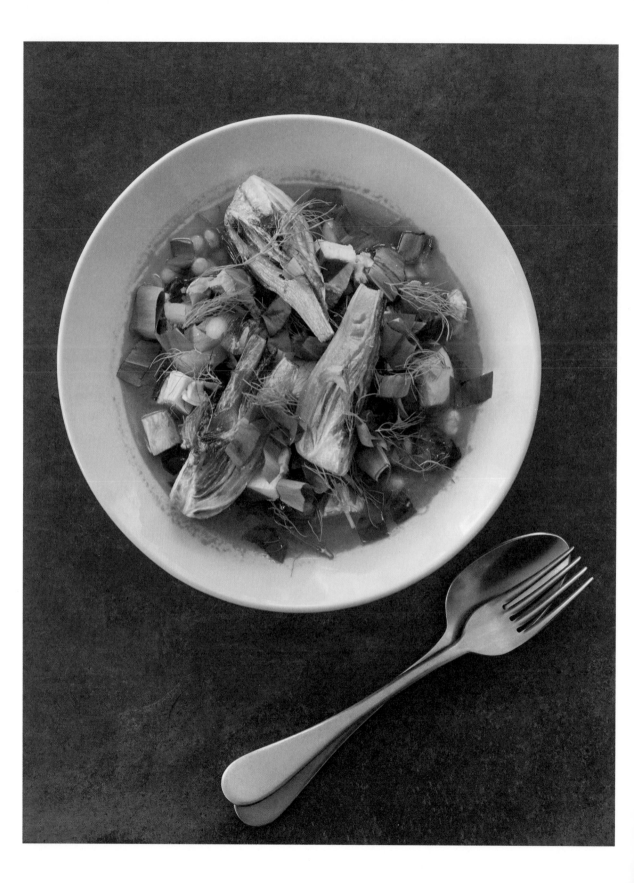

I make this every week at home, using sweet rather than spicy chorizo. The kids love the flavour and it's easy and quick to prepare, especially if you have some leftover roast chicken in the refrigerator. I finish this with some chopped wild garlic leaves; if you can't get them or they are out of season, rocket (arugula) or watercress gives the dish a similar nice peppery finish. Also, although delicious, the caramelised fennel wedges aren't essential; if you prefer to keep things simple, you can leave them out.

CHICKEN, CHORIZO AND FENNEL STEW

SERVES 4

2–3 tbsp olive oil

2 garlic cloves, crushed

1 tsp crushed fennel seeds

1 onion, diced

2 fennel bulbs: 1 diced; 1 chopped into wedges (optional); fronds reserved, if possible

4 x 100g (3¾oz) fresh chorizo sausages (sweet or spicy according to preference), skinned and broken into small chunks

1 x 400g (14oz) can crushed tomatoes

200ml (scant 1 cup) chicken stock

1 x 400g (14oz) can white beans

400g (14oz) cooked chicken (breast or leg meat), chopped

a handful of chopped wild garlic (or rocket /arugula or watercress)

sea salt and freshly ground black pepper, to taste

1. Heat 2 tablespoons of the olive oil in a saucepan over a medium heat, add the garlic and fennel seeds and cook, stirring until the garlic begins to lightly colour. Add the onion and diced fennel, then reduce the heat and sweat for 5 minutes. Add the chorizo chunks, increase the heat slightly and fry for 5 minutes until the chorizo, onion and fennel have begun to colour slightly. Add the crushed tomatoes and chicken stock and boil for about 15 minutes until reduced by half. Be careful: if molten tomato begins firing around the kitchen, just reduce the temperature a little until it stops.

2. If you are serving the caramelised fennel wedges, heat the remaining tablespoon of olive oil in a frying pan and gently fry the fennel wedges for about 5 minutes on each side until they are softened and golden all over.

3. Add the white beans and chicken to the stew, bring back to a simmer and cook for a further 10 minutes to allow everything to get to know one another. Season to taste.

4. Serve the stew in a deep serving plate, topped with a few of the caramelised fennel wedges, some chopped wild garlic and the fennel fronds.

The night before a race, it's better to stick with a dish you have eaten before, and this is one of my go-to pre-race suppers. The quinoa supplies the carbs you need for fuel before the big push of a race and the addition of fresh herbs makes the entire meal much lighter. The result is a vibrant dish that should leave you light on your feet and ready to go at the start line.

ROAST CHICKEN WITH QUINOA TABBOULEH AND CHICORY

SERVES 4

1 x 1.5kg (3½lb) chicken (preferably organic)

extra-virgin olive oil, for drizzling

2 tbsp za'atar

salt and freshly ground black pepper, to taste

feta cheese, to serve

2 heads of red chicory (red Belgian endive), trimmed, leaves separated, to serve

Greek or Turkish yogurt, to serve

FOR THE QUINOA TABBOULEH:

200g (7oz) quinoa

1 small red onion, finely diced

2 tomatoes, deseeded and finely diced

½ cucumber, finely diced

½ garlic clove, crushed

a handful each of parsley, mint, dill, basil, rocket (arugula) and fresh coriander (cilantro), coarsely chopped

juice of 1 lemon

2 tbsp white wine vinegar

a pinch of dried Turkish chilli flakes (optional)

extra-virgin olive oil

salt and freshly ground black pepper, to taste

1. Preheat the oven to 220°C/425°F/Gas 7.

2. To spatchcock the chicken, place the bird breast-side down, legs facing you. Use a pair of strong kitchen scissors to cut along either side of the backbone (avoid cutting through the meat connecting the legs to the backbone – these are the 'oysters' and are the best bit). Remove the backbone, turn the bird over and press on the breastbone with the heel of your hand to flatten the meat out. Place the chicken, skin-side up, in a roasting pan, drizzle with olive oil and season with salt, pepper and za'atar. Roast for about 40 minutes until the skin is golden and the leg juices run clear when pierced. Allow to rest for 5–10 minutes.

3. Meanwhile, for the quinoa tabbouleh, cook the quinoa in a saucepan of boiling salted water, according to the packet instructions. Remove from the heat and allow to cool slightly.

4. Mix together the other tabbouleh ingredients in a large bowl, along with a very generous glug of olive oil, and salt and pepper, to taste. Mix in the cooled quinoa until well combined.

5. Spread the tabbouleh over a large platter, crumble over the feta and place the chicken on top. Serve with the chicory, lightly dressed with olive oil, and Greek yogurt on the side. Let everyone dig in.

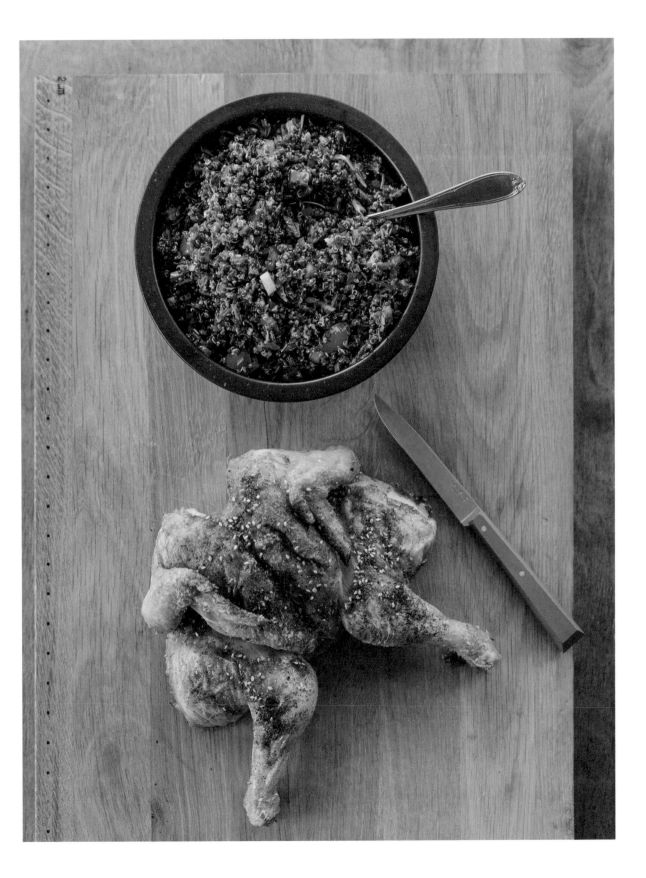

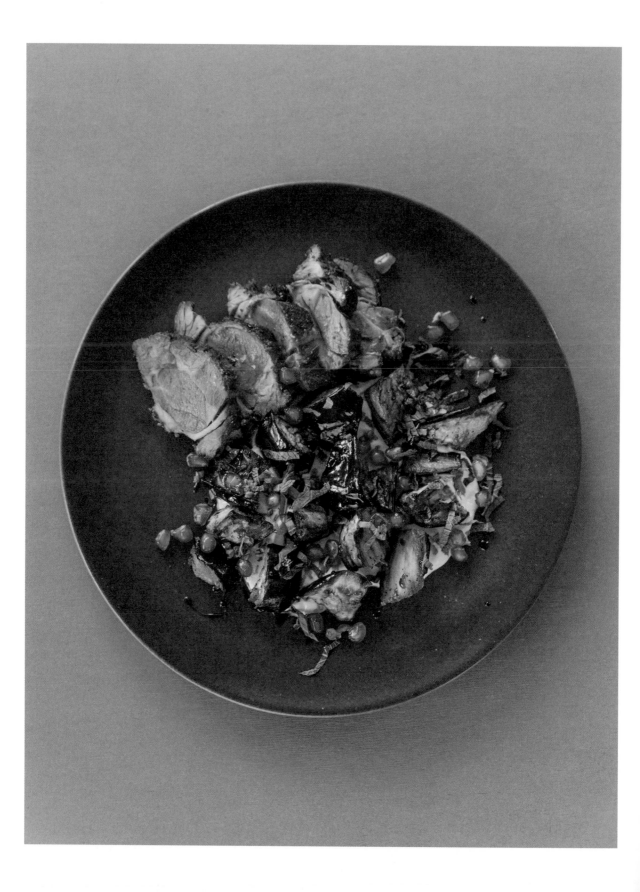

Lamb rump is a great cut of meat, not often used, but the fat content gives it a fantastic rich flavour and it is high in iron and a rich source of protein. Sheep do not respond well to bad farming practices, they are happiest left alone in the field grazing not packed into pens, so the likelihood of the meat coming from an ethical source is much higher than with beef or pork. This dish is best when it's served still a little pink, but if you prefer your meat well-done, the rump is a good cut to use as the fat keeps it from drying out.

SPICED LAMB WITH ROAST AUBERGINE, TAHINI YOGURT AND POMEGRANATE

SERVES 4

1 tbsp cumin seeds

1 tbsp coriander seeds

½ tsp dried chilli flakes

600g (1⅓lb) lamb rump, cut into 4 pieces

2 aubergines (eggplants), trimmed and cut into 2cm (¾in) pieces

4 tbsp extra-virgin olive oil

200g (7oz) Tahini Yogurt (see p.30)

3 tbsp pomegranate molasses

seeds of ½ pomegranate

a handful of fresh mint, coarsely chopped

sea salt and freshly ground black pepper, to taste

1. Preheat the oven to 180°C/350°F/Gas 4.

2. In a pestle and mortar, pound the cumin seeds, coriander seeds and chilli flakes with ½ teaspoon salt and a few grindings of black pepper until well crushed. Coat the lamb pieces with the spice mix and set aside for at least 30 minutes to come to room temperature.

3. In a roasting pan, mix the aubergines with 3 tablespoons of the olive oil, then season with salt and roast for 20–25 minutes until softened and golden brown.

4. Meanwhile, heat the remaining olive oil in a cast-iron frying pan over a high heat and sear the spiced lamb for 2 minutes on each side until dark golden brown. Transfer the pan to the oven (or place the meat in a roasting pan) and roast for 10–12 minutes until medium rare or 55°C (131°F) on a meat thermometer. Remove from the oven and allow to rest for at least 5 minutes.

5. To serve, spoon the tahini yogurt onto serving plates and top with the roasted aubergine. Drizzle over the pomegranate molasses and scatter over the pomegranate seeds and chopped mint. Slice the lamb against the grain and arrange on each plate.

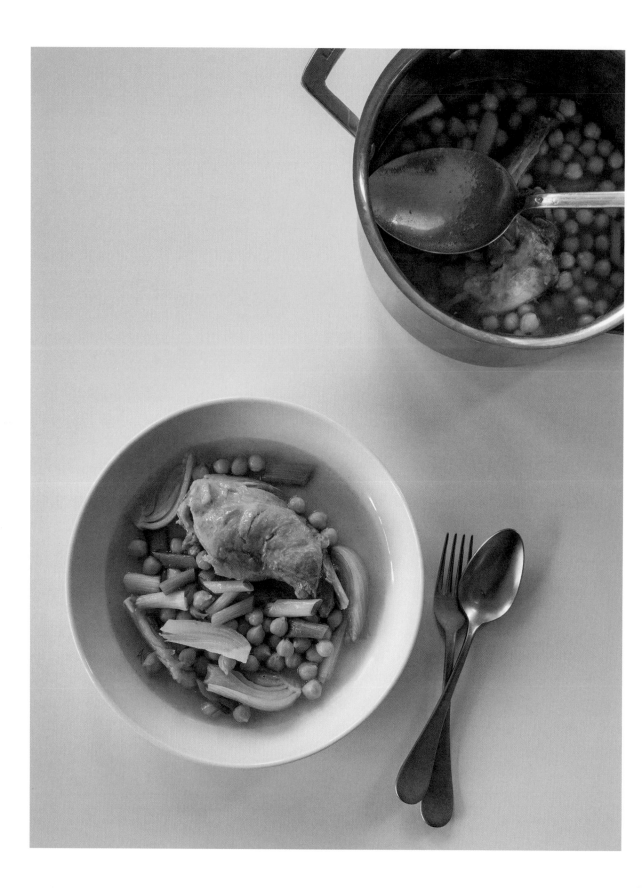

Naturally low in fat and high in iron and protein, rabbit is a great alternative to other meats and I highly recommend giving it a go. I love the mild flavour and, partnered with fennel, fresh garlic and good olive oil, it's a real treat – one of my favourites.

Ask your local butcher to get you farmed rabbit for this recipe, as they are larger and much more tender. Wild rabbit is equally delicious, but has much stronger flavour and needs a delicate hand when it comes to cooking. You only need the front and hind legs for this recipe. If you can't buy the legs separately, buy two whole rabbits and ask your butcher to joint them – you could save the saddles for a future meal.

BRAISED RABBIT WITH FENNEL, GREEN GARLIC AND CHICKPEAS

SERVES 4

8 rabbit legs (4 front and 4 hind legs)

4 tbsp extra-virgin olive oil, plus extra to serve

2 tsp fennel seeds, lightly crushed

2 fresh green garlic bulbs, coarsely chopped (or 1 regular garlic bulb, unpeeled, halved widthways)

3 fennel bulbs: 1 coarsely chopped; 2 cut into wedges

1 white onion, coarsely chopped

1 glass of dry sherry or white wine

2 litres (8 cups) chicken stock

1 x 400g (14oz) can chickpeas

a bunch of spring onions (scallions), coarsely chopped

sea salt and freshly ground black pepper, to taste

bread, to serve

1. Preheat the oven to 120°C/250°F/Gas ½. Season the rabbit legs with salt.

2. In a large ovenproof pot or casserole with a lid, gently heat the olive oil over a medium heat, then add the crushed fennel seeds and the rabbit legs. Sear for 2 minutes on each side until lightly coloured, then add the garlic, chopped fennel and white onion.

3. Sweat down the vegetables for 5 minutes, then add the sherry or wine and simmer until almost all the wine has evaporated. Add the chicken stock and bring to a simmer, then cover with the lid and place in the oven for 1½–2 hours until the rabbit meat is beginning to fall off the bone.

4. Remove the rabbit legs from the pot with a slotted spoon, trying not to break them up too much, and set aside. Strain the cooking liquid, discarding the vegetables (this might seem wasteful, but all their flavour is now in the stock), then return the stock to the pot. Bring to a gentle simmer, then add the chickpeas and fennel wedges and simmer for 15 minutes until the fennel is tender. Add the chopped spring onions and return the rabbit legs to the pot, then simmer for a further 10 minutes so that all the ingredients get to know one another. Season with salt and pepper.

5. Serve with a little extra drizzle of olive oil and some good bread.

I don't eat too much red meat, but from time to time I really do enjoy a steak. Flank steak is from the lower chest of the cow and not a common cut – it can become tough if overcooked and, more importantly, not sliced against the grain – but the flavour is much deeper than fillet steak or sirloin. This means it's more satisfying when you have a smaller portion, plus the extra chewing is good for the jaw muscles!

The fermented red cabbage and labneh are both probiotics and the raw onion in the slaw is a prebiotic; all three will help with the growth of healthy gut bacteria.

FLANK STEAK WITH FERMENTED RED SLAW, LABNEH AND SWEET POTATO WEDGES

SERVES 4

2 large sweet potatoes, peeled and chopped into wedges

about 4 tbsp extra-virgin olive oil

400g (14oz) Red Sauerkraut (see p.197) or sliced red cabbage

1 small red onion, very thinly sliced

600g (1⅓lb) flank steak (remove from the refrigerator 30 minutes before cooking)

1 tbsp butter

200g (7oz) Labneh (see p.24)

sea salt and freshly ground black pepper, to taste

1. Preheat the oven to 180°C/350°F/Gas 4.

2. In a roasting pan, coat the sweet potato wedges with 2 tablespoons of the olive oil and a pinch of salt. Roast for 25–30 minutes until golden brown and crisp. Remove from the oven and drain any excess fat on kitchen paper.

3. In a large mixing bowl, blend the red sauerkraut or cabbage and sliced red onion with a glug of olive oil. Taste and season with salt, if necessary.

4. Season the steak with salt and plenty of black pepper. Heat a cast-iron frying pan until smoking hot, then add 1 tablespoon of the olive oil and the steak and cook for 1 minute. Add the butter and cook for a further 2 minutes, then flip the steak over to cook for another 2 minutes. Remove the steak from the pan and allow to rest for 5 minutes – it should be cooked no more than medium and still nice and pink in the middle.

5. Slice the steak against the grain and serve with a spoonful of labneh and the red slaw, with the roasted sweet potatoes on the side. If you like, this is also great with some fresh coriander (cilantro) and fresh chillies, served with small corn tortillas.

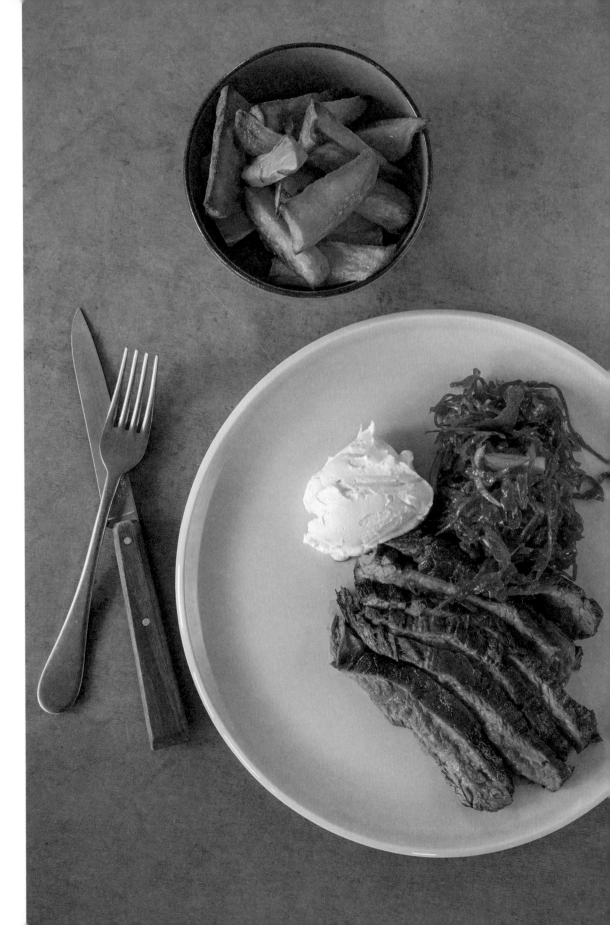

I cook this often – it's delicious, very quick and easy to prepare and the kids love it. I always add chilli flakes at the end to keep it child friendly, but if you want some extra kick add a teaspoon of chilli powder to the spice paste.

COD WITH CURRIED COCONUT LEEKS

SERVES 4

2 tbsp coconut oil

2 leeks, trimmed, washed and sliced

1 x 400ml (1²/₃ cups) can coconut milk

4 x 150g (5oz) pieces of cod fillet

sea salt, to taste

a handful of fresh coriander (cilantro), leaves picked, to garnish

dried chilli flakes, to taste (optional)

cooked brown rice, to serve

FOR THE SPICE PASTE:

½ tsp salt

2 garlic cloves, peeled

1 tsp curry powder (as hot as you like)

½ tsp fenugreek seeds

½ tsp coriander seeds

½ tsp ground turmeric

1. First, make the spice paste. In a pestle and mortar, crush the salt, garlic and spices to a paste.

2. Melt half of the coconut oil in a saucepan over a medium heat, add the spice paste and cook for 2 minutes, then add the leeks and sweat down for a couple of minutes until they begin to soften. Pour in the coconut milk, bring to a simmer and cook for 10–15 minutes until the sauce is thick.

3. Meanwhile, heat a frying pan until just smoking hot, then reduce the heat to medium and add the remaining coconut oil. Season the cod fillets with a little sea salt and place in the pan. Cook for 5–6 minutes on each side until the flesh is a lovely golden colour and flakes apart.

4. Serve the cod and curried leek sauce with brown rice, garnished with fresh coriander and a pinch of chilli flakes, if desired.

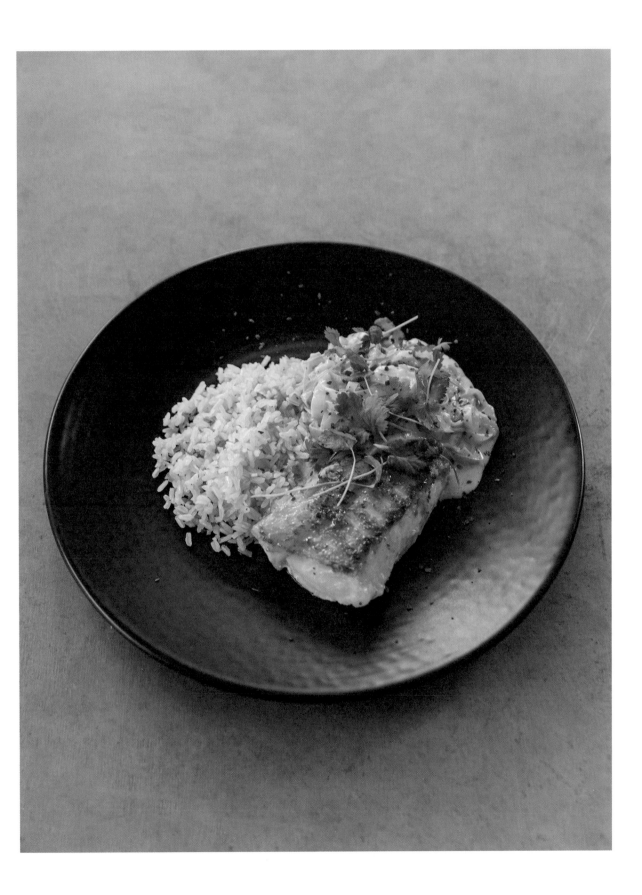

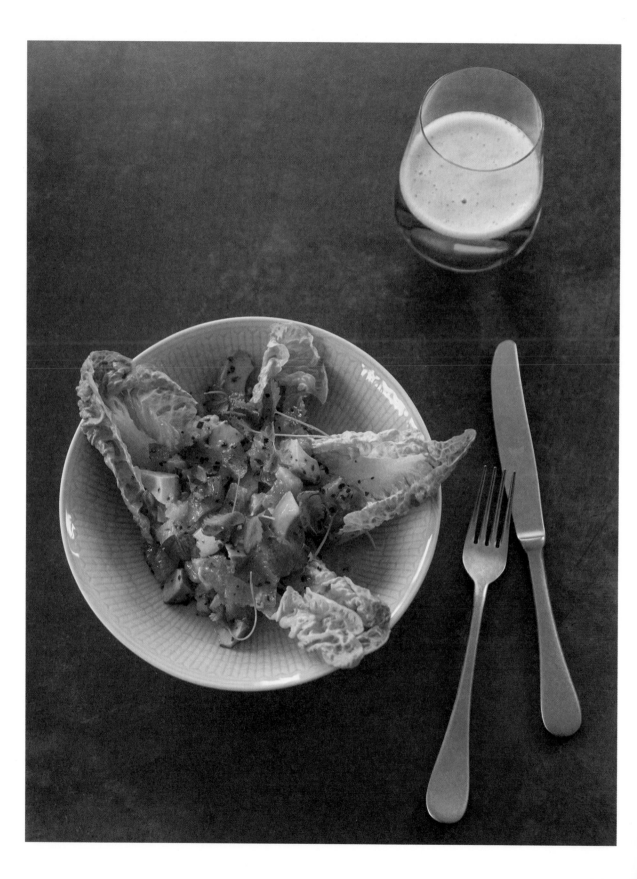

Ceviche originated in Peru and there is evidence that it has been eaten there for more than two thousand years. The raw fish is 'cooked' by the addition of citrus juice instead of heat. I always briefly freeze any fish that I'm going to eat raw, cure or use in a ceviche, just to be sure that any parasites are killed off. Chefs are often a bit snobby when it comes to freezing products, but in this case I think it's better to be safe than sorry. Always use wild salmon or farmed salmon with the MSC mark, to be sure it has been sustainably fished. You can replace the salmon with trout, mackerel or even white fish, such as cod or haddock.

SALMON AND CITRUS CEVICHE

SERVES 4

600g (1⅓lb) fresh salmon fillet, skinned and pin bones removed (defrosted if previously frozen)

½ tsp sea salt, or more to taste

1 pink grapefruit

1 blood orange

juice of 1 lime, or more to taste

1 romaine lettuce, trimmed and leaves pulled apart

2 avocados, flesh only, chopped into 1cm (²/₅in) pieces

a handful of fresh coriander (cilantro) leaves

dried chilli flakes, for sprinkling (optional)

1. Cut the salmon into 1cm (²/₅in) pieces, transfer to a mixing bowl and season with the salt. Set aside.

2. With a sharp knife, cut the top and bottom off the grapefruit – this gives you a firm base to stand the fruit on. Following the shape of the fruit, cut off the peel, removing as much of the white rind as you can. Next, cut each segment away from the core, by carefully slicing between the membranes. Repeat with the blood orange. Cut each segment in half, then add to the bowl with the salmon, along with the lime juice. Mix gently so as not to break up the citrus fruit. Taste for seasoning – it may need a touch more salt or lime juice.

3. Divide the salad leaves among 4 serving plates and top each with a large spoonful of the salmon ceviche and the chopped avocado. Finish with a sprinkling of fresh coriander and dried chilli flakes, if wished.

Mackerel is my favourite fish. It's best in early spring and absolutely must be eaten as fresh as possible. High in protein and rich in omega 3 fatty acids, it is robust enough to handle heavy spicing, as in this dish or the Smoked Mackerel Kedgeree on p.37, and it also makes for fantastic sushi or crudo.

DEVILLED MACKEREL WITH KOHLRABI AND CUCUMBER SALAD

SERVES 4

100g (3¾oz) salted butter, softened

2 tsp cayenne pepper

½ tsp dried chilli flakes

2 tsp muscovado sugar

2 tsp ground coriander

1 tsp English mustard powder

2 tsp Dijon mustard

2 tsp red wine vinegar

juice of 1 lemon

4 whole mackerel (about 300g (11oz) each), gutted, cleaned and trimmed

1 kohlrabi

1 cucumber

a handful of curly parsley, chopped

a drizzle of extra-virgin olive oil

salt and freshly ground black pepper, to taste

300g (11oz) Greek yogurt, to serve

lemon wedges, to serve

1. Preheat the grill to the highest setting.

2. Mix the butter with the cayenne pepper, chilli flakes, sugar, ground coriander, mustards, vinegar, half of the lemon juice and a little salt and pepper. Rub all over the mackerel, inside and out.

3. Peel the kohlrabi and slice as thinly as possible (a mandoline is great for this, but do mind your fingers). Slice the cucumber in half lengthways and cut into 5mm (¹/₅in)- thick half-moons. Place the kohlrabi and cucumber in a bowl and dress with the chopped parsley, a drizzle of olive oil and the remaining lemon juice. Season with a pinch of salt and set aside.

4. Place the mackerel onto the rack of the grill pan and grill for 4–5 minutes on each side or until cooked through.

5. Serve the mackerel with the kohlrabi and cucumber salad, with Greek yogurt and lemon wedges on the side.

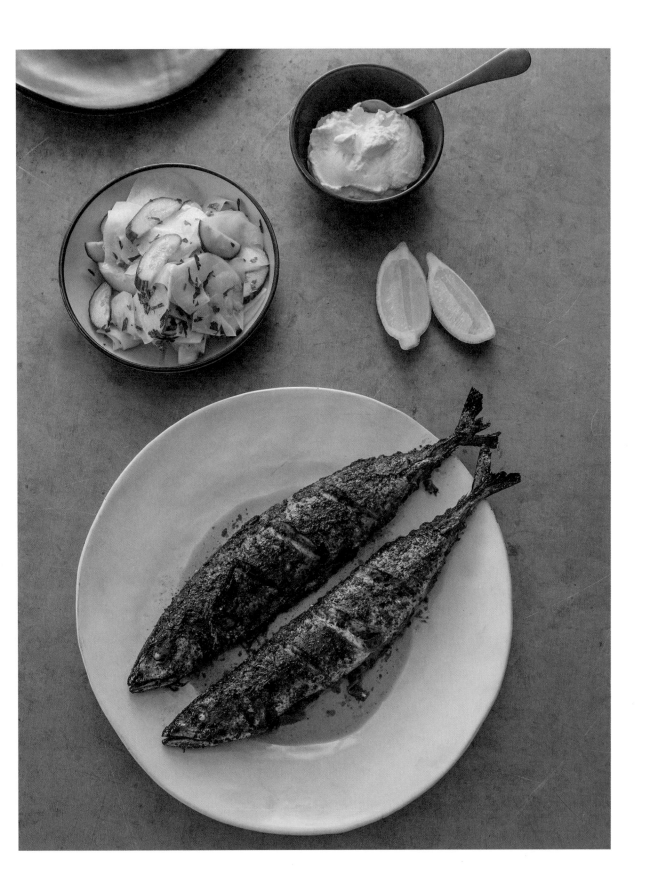

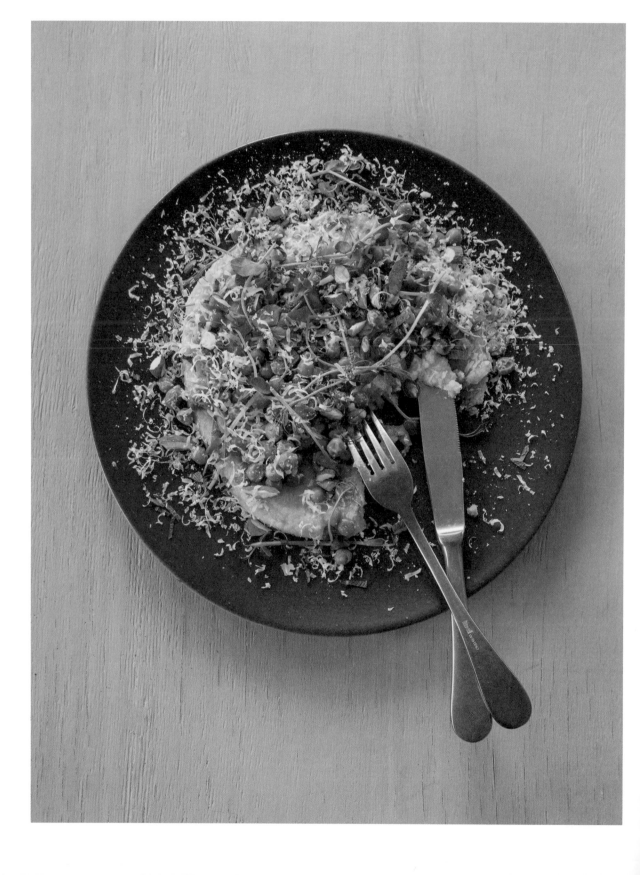

This is a classic Italian flavour combination. There's something comforting about a big bowl of creamy polenta and sometimes after a long run that's just what you need! Polenta is rich in dietary fibre and a good source of gluten-free carbohydrates; also, the forty-five minutes of stirring is good strength training for your arms.

POLENTA WITH PEAS, PECORINO AND ALMONDS

SERVES 4

150ml (²/₃ cup) milk

600ml (2½ cups) water, plus about 3 tbsp

½ tsp salt

150g (5oz) coarse polenta

50g (2oz) butter

75g (2½oz) Pecorino cheese, grated

1 tbsp extra-virgin olive oil

1 shallot, finely chopped

200g (7oz) fresh podded peas (or use frozen)

a handful of pea shoots

a few fresh mint sprigs, chopped

80g (3oz) almonds, coarsely chopped

freshly ground black pepper, to taste

1. In a large, heavy saucepan, bring the milk, 600ml (2½ cups) water and salt to the boil. Once it is boiling, add the polenta, whisking continuously. Cook, stirring, for 1–2 minutes until it thickens. Reduce the heat to low and cook for a further 35–45 minutes, stirring well every 4–5 minutes to prevent sticking until the polenta begins to come away from the sides of the saucepan. Stir in the butter and one-third of the Pecorino cheese.

2. Meanwhile, heat the olive oil in a separate saucepan over a low heat, add the shallot and sweat for 2 minutes, then add the peas along with about 3 tablespoons water. Bring to the boil and cook until the water has almost evaporated. The peas should be just cooked and glazed with the remaining liquid.

3. Serve the polenta on a large serving dish or individual plates, topped with the peas, pea shoots, chopped mint and almonds. Finish with the remaining grated Pecorino and a grinding of black pepper.

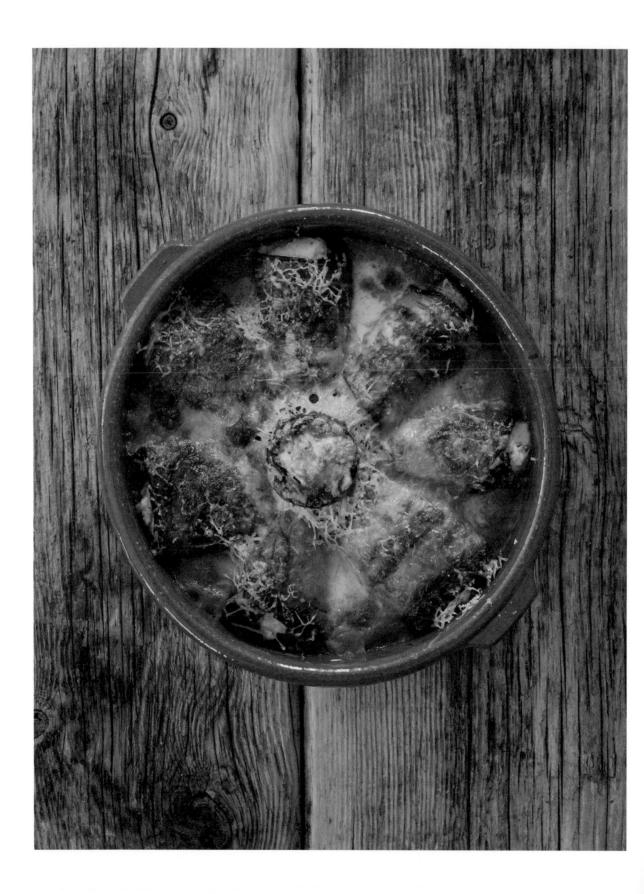

Aubergines, tomatoes and peppers are all are rich in potassium, which helps lower blood pressure, improves muscle function and is one of the essential minerals for our electrolyte balance (the complicated process of sending the liquids we take in to the places in the body that need it). They are also three ingredients that are almost always delicious when served together.

AUBERGINE AND RICOTTA INVOLTINI

SERVES 4

2-3 medium aubergines (eggplants), stems removed

olive oil, for frying

100ml (scant ½ cup) double cream

50g (2oz) Parmesan cheese, grated

sea salt and freshly ground black pepper, to taste

peppery salad dressed with red wine vinegar and olive oil, to serve (optional)

FOR THE TOMATO SAUCE:

3 tbsp olive oil

3 garlic cloves, peeled and smashed

1 yellow onion, finely chopped

1 red pepper, deseeded and finely chopped

1 tsp red wine vinegar, plus extra to taste

1 x 400g (14oz) can chopped tomatoes

FOR THE STUFFING:

250g (9oz) ricotta cheese

3-4 slices of 4-day-old bread, blitzed into breadcrumbs

zest of 1 lemon

3-4 sage leaves, chopped

1. For the sauce, heat the oil in a saucepan over a medium-high heat, add the garlic and a few grindings of black pepper and cook for 1 minute until the garlic starts to colour. Add the onion and red pepper and sweat for 5 minutes until softened and just starting to colour. Add the vinegar, cook for 1 minute, then add the tomatoes. Rinse the can out with a little water and add that to the saucepan, increase the heat and bring to the boil. Reduce the heat and simmer for 20–30 minutes until the sauce is thick and the vegetables have broken down a little. Season with salt and a little more vinegar, to taste.

2. For the stuffing, mix the ricotta in a bowl with the breadcrumbs, lemon zest and sage leaves, and season well. Set aside.

3. Meanwhile, slice the aubergines length-ways about 7mm (¼in) thick; you should have at least 16 slices. Heat a frying pan over a medium heat and pour in a generous amount of oil. Fry 3–4 slices at a time, for 2–3 minutes on each side until softened and slightly coloured. Drain on kitchen paper. Repeat with the remaining slices.

4. Preheat the oven to 190°C/375°F/Gas 5.

5. Pour the sauce into a large baking dish. Place a spoonful of the stuffing at one end of each aubergine slice and roll it up around the stuffing. Place the rolls on top of the sauce, seam-side down. Spoon the cream over the rolls and top with the grated Parmesan. Bake for 20–25 minutes until the rolls are golden brown and the sauce is bubbling. This is great with a peppery salad of rocket and watercress, dressed with red wine vinegar and olive oil.

This a handy recipe, ready in the time it takes to boil the pasta. The cavolo nero is full of iron, which is something that long-distance runners often struggle to get enough of in their diet. Any leftover pesto can be kept in the refrigerator for a few days – just put it into a small jar and cover the top with some olive oil.

SPAGHETTI WITH CAVOLO NERO AND WALNUT PESTO

SERVES 4

350g (12oz) dried spaghetti (or any pasta will do)

1 head of cavolo nero (about 200g /7oz), leaves picked from the stalks and rinsed

100g (3¾oz) toasted walnuts

80g (3oz) Parmesan cheese, finely grated, plus extra to serve

1 small garlic clove, peeled

a pinch of crushed dried chilli flakes (optional)

50ml (¼ cup) extra-virgin olive oil, or more as needed

salt and freshly ground black pepper, to taste

1. Bring a large saucepan of salted water to the boil, add the pasta and cook according to the packet instructions, or until slightly al dente.

2. Meanwhile, put the cavolo nero, walnuts, Parmesan, garlic and chilli flakes into a food processor, then add a pinch of salt and a grinding or two of black pepper. Process, slowly pouring in the olive oil through the feed tube, until well blended to a dark green paste. Taste to check seasoning, and adjust if necessary.

3. Drain the pasta and stir through the pesto while it is still warm. Serve with extra Parmesan on the side.

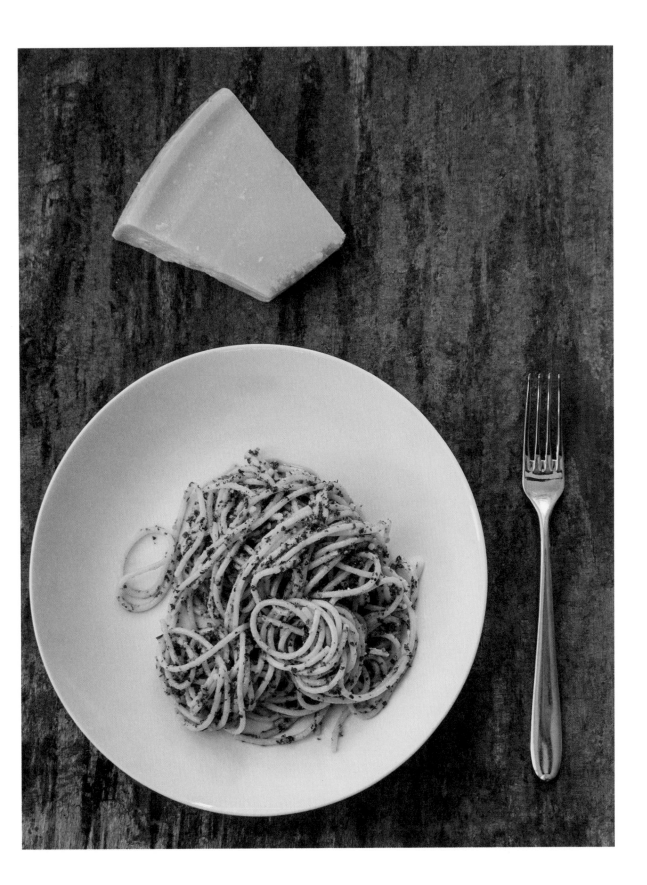

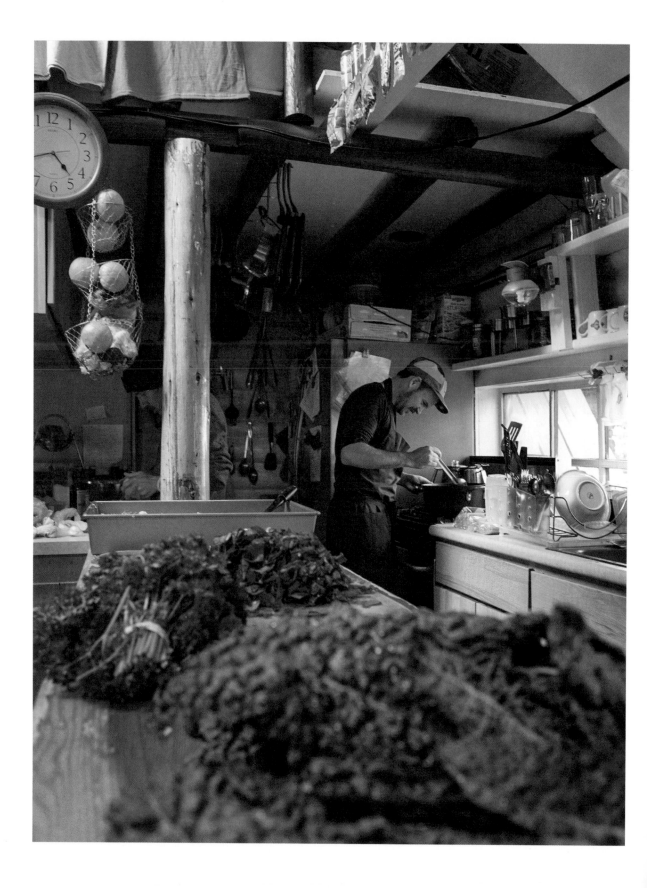

What to serve to a lodge full of hungry hikers? Being 6 miles (10km) from town, guests at Barr Camp have no choice but to eat what is served to them, but it could make for an uncomfortable evening if it were not well received. Knowing that pasta is a mainstay on the menu at Barr Camp, I opted to stick with that, but instead of a red sauce I decided to mix it up and use some of the wonderful greens available in the market in town: green kale, cavolo nero and rainbow chard, with garlic, olive oil and lots of chopped roasted almonds. Thankfully, it went down well and, served alongside Barr Camp's famous garlic bread (see p.193) and a roaring fire, it was a great evening.

PASTA WITH MIXED GREENS AND ROASTED ALMONDS

SERVES 4

400g (14oz) dried spaghetti

5 tbsp extra-virgin olive oil

1 large onion, diced

4 garlic cloves, peeled and sliced

400g (14oz) mixed greens (kale, cavolo nero, rainbow chard), chopped

200g (7oz) roasted almonds, chopped

a handful of flat-leaf parsley, coarsely chopped

100g (3¾oz) Parmesan cheese, grated, plus extra to serve

sea salt and freshly ground black pepper, to taste

1. Bring a large saucepan of salted water to the boil and cook the pasta according to the packet instructions.

2. Meanwhile, heat the olive oil in a large sauté pan over a medium heat, add the onion and garlic and sweat for 5–6 minutes until softened. Add the greens and ½ teaspoon salt, then reduce the heat and cook for 15–20 minutes until the greens are soft (they will have lost some of their bright green colour, but the flavour will have developed and become almost sweet). Fold in the cooked pasta, roasted almonds, parsley and Parmesan. Season with a little more salt and plenty of black pepper, to taste.

3. Serve with a little extra grated Parmesan sprinkled on top.

On the Trail with:

Zach Miller

Colorado, USA

WHEN I THINK about trail running, the first place that comes to mind is Colorado – home to some of the world's most iconic 100-mile trails, such as Leadville, which was written about in the book *Born to Run*, and the notoriously beautiful and brutal Hardrock 100. A who's who of elite mountain runners live locally. This is not surprising, since half of the state is covered in spectacular mountain ranges and even the flatland plains have an elevation of over 1000 metres (3300 feet) above sea level; it's a runner's paradise.

I was lucky enough to be invited to stay and cook with local ultra runner Zack Miller. Zach blasted on to the trail running scene in 2013 with back-to-back wins at two of the most competitive races in America, the JFK 50 and the Lake Sonoma 50. His go-for-broke running style has won him

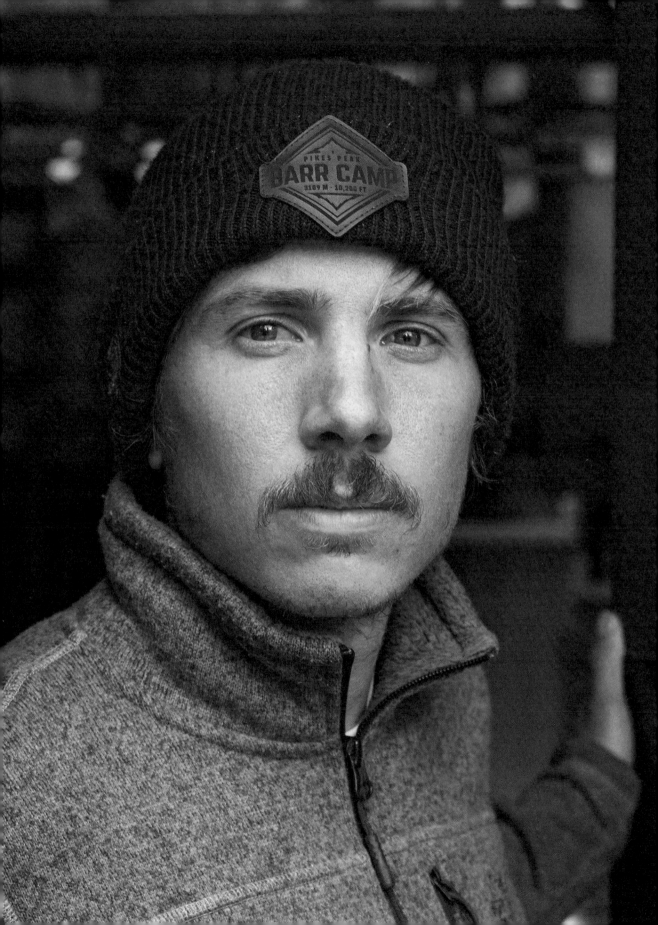

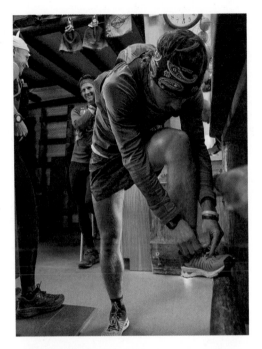
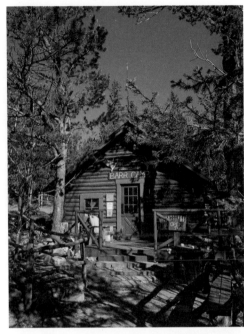
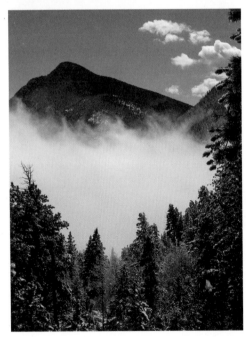
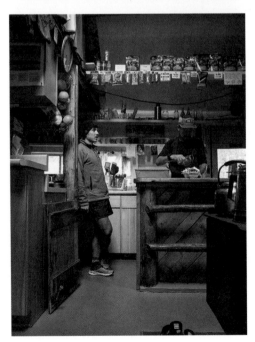

ZACH MILLER

«We are asking a lot from our bodies, so we need to be mindful of what we put back into them.»

————————

fans all over the world. I met him at his home and workplace, Barr Camp, an off-grid hikers' refuge located halfway up Pikes Peak in Manitou Springs. Here, Zach and his colleagues, Reagan and Lonnie, are caretakers and their daily tasks vary from chopping firewood to cooking breakfast and dinner, and even mountain rescue.

The camp is 3109 metres (10,200 feet) above sea level and the only way to get up to it is a 6-mile (10km) uphill hike on the iconic Barr Trail. In good conditions, this would normally be a three-hour hike from the town, but on my visit we had the first snow of the year the evening before, so – although beautiful – that made the hike a little trickier!

After cooking nightly suppers for up to 50 guests at the camp for the last couple of years, it's no surprise that Zach is a very good cook, fuelled by a real love for food. I could see by watching him prepare our dinner that evening that cooking is not a chore for him. He takes his food and nutrition seriously – a necessity, since he needs to really pack in the calories to supplement all the training. He eats mostly wholefoods and few processed ingredients, but nothing is off limits and he allows

himself the occasional fast-food feast. 'Eating is training,' as Zach puts it. 'We are asking a lot from our bodies, so we need to be mindful of what we put back into them.'

A handful of times a year, The Pikes Peak COG Railway brings up basic stocks (pasta, canned tomatoes, oats, etc.) to a point just 1.5 miles (2.4km) from the camp, but all fresh food must be hiked in from the town below. This can pose some problems, but as the 12-mile (20km) loop to and from town is regularly used for training, Zach's packs are often filled with lots of bananas, blueberries, spinach and red meat.

The following morning, Zach invited me to join him for a run up towards the summit of Pikes Peak. After a big breakfast of pancakes (see p.38 for the Barr Camp recipe), peanut butter and coffee, we set off uphill at a steady pace. Zach chatted away comfortably, telling stories of the local area and of his experiences of running in his little corner of the Rockies. However, the altitude hit me after only a few hundred metres! We started out at about 3000 metres (9,843 feet) above sea level and were heading upwards. As Zach gently

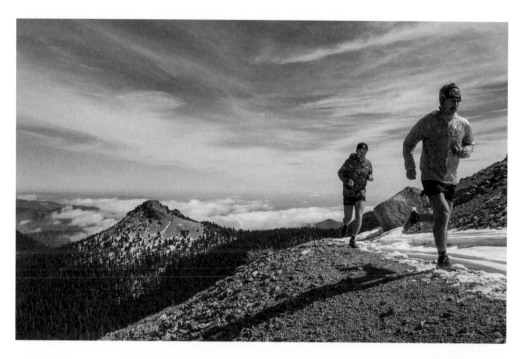

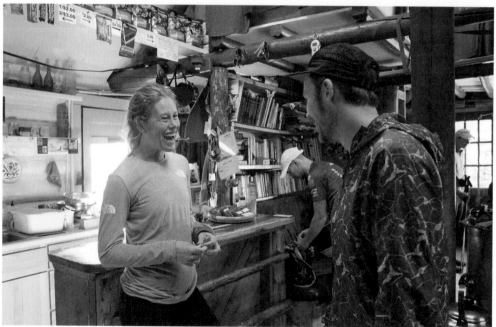

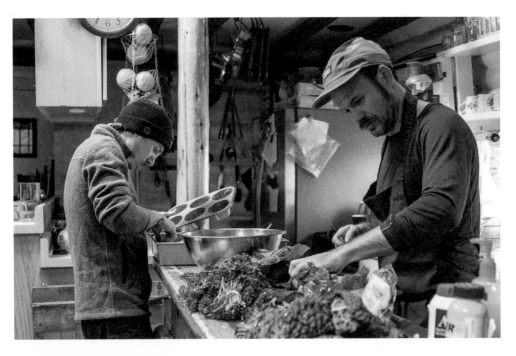

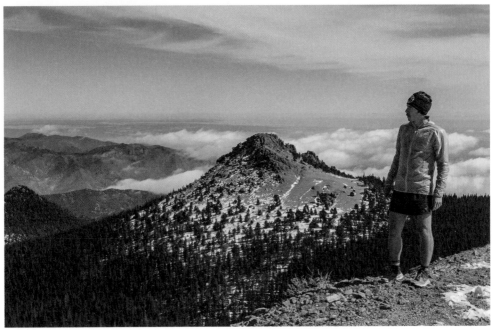

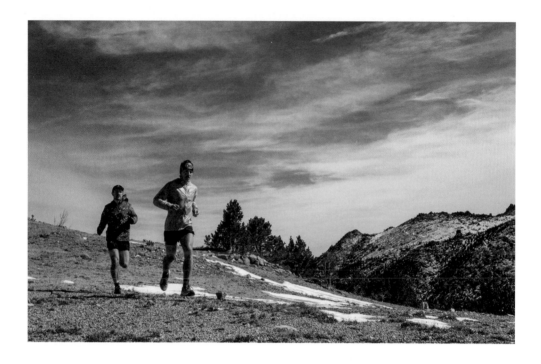

jogged on, chatting away, my responses turned to grunts and splutters. After 4 miles (6.4km) we reached a plateau (at 3800 metres/12,467 feet, I later learned) and I gestured for Zach to run on. After a few minutes of recovery, I headed back to camp with a new-found admiration for anyone who can move so well at this elevation.

That evening, I cooked for the 20 or so hungry hikers who were staying at the camp. I made spaghetti with kale, rainbow chard, cavolo nero and roasted almonds (see p.137); a simple dish, but packed with flavour and all the nutrients needed after a big day in the mountains. Zach assisted me and gave me a few tips on how to make the legendary Barr Camp Switchback Garlic Bread (see p.193).

There was a family from Texas, a Romanian university lecturer, a couple of Zach's friends who happened to be visiting from Pennsylvania and a few local runners from the town, all sitting around the fire eating together, and there was a real sense of communal spirit. We finished up with a simple Apple Crumble (see p.164), a dessert that is always well received, especially by people who've had a long day on their feet. We turned in for the night, full to bursting and exhausted.

The following morning, Zach was already in the kitchen when I woke up – the campers needed

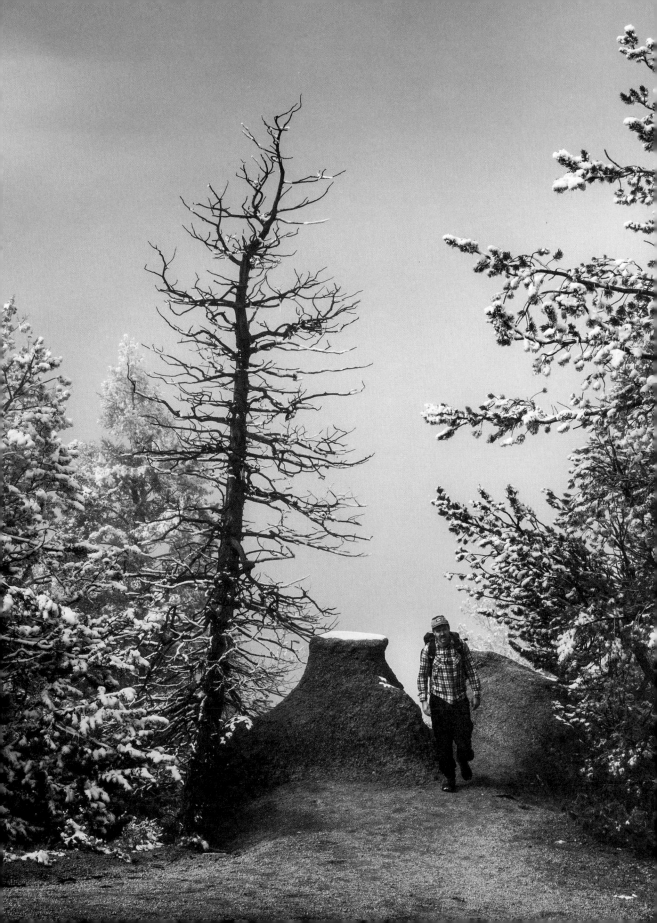

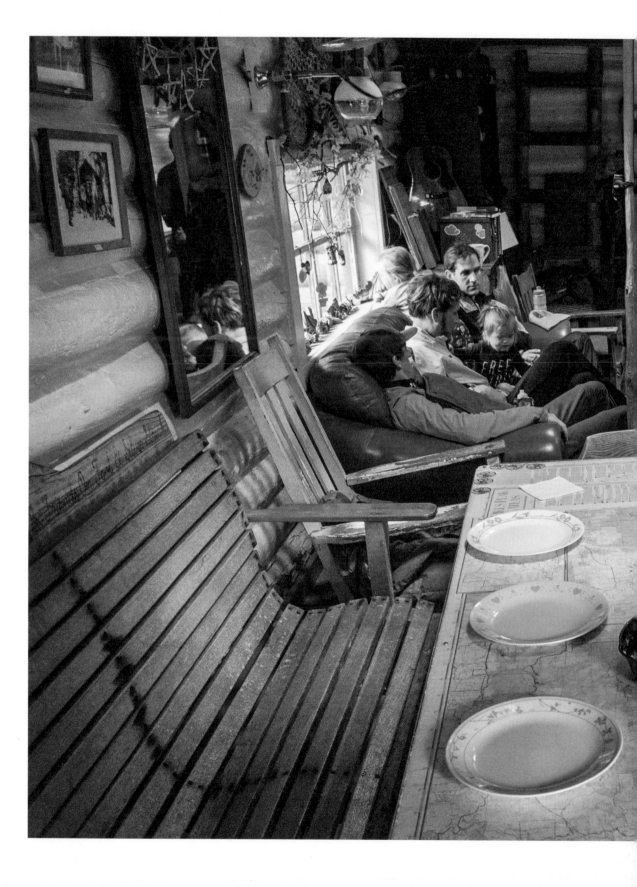

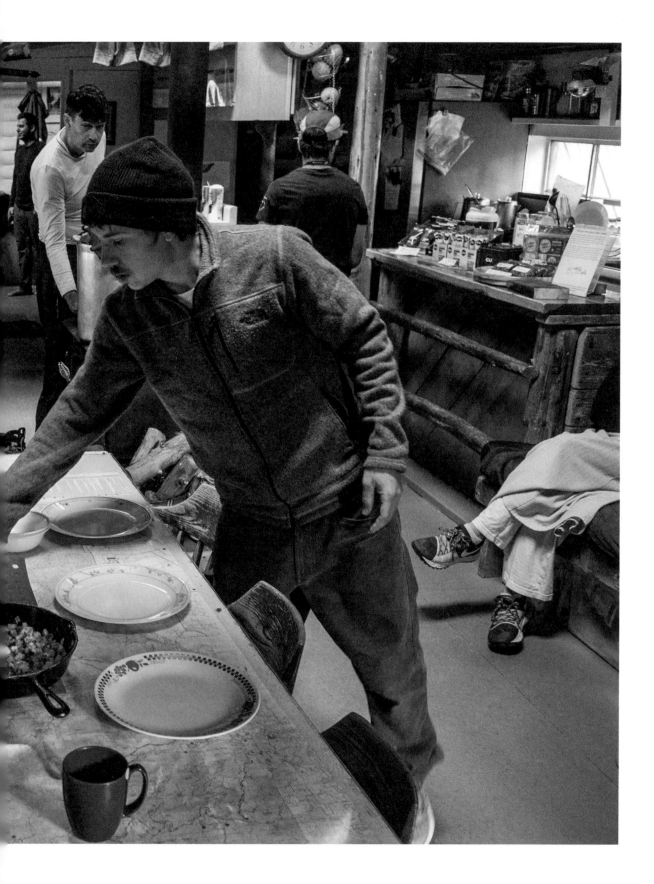

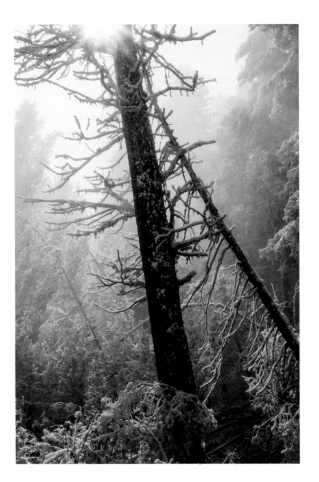

feeding! He made a change from the usual pancakes and instead cooked baked oatmeal (see p.26), a Pennsylvanian classic, served straight from the oven with cold milk. It's a cross between a flapjack and ordinary porridge, packed with dried berries and lightly spiced with cinnamon. It was a great way to start the day, especially as I knew I shortly had to run the 6 miles (10km) back down to town.

As I was about to head off, Zach was lacing up his shoes once again to run to the summit of Pikes Peak, at 4300 metres (14,115 feet), that was 1200 metres (4000 feet) higher and usually a day's hike from Barr Camp. His running partner was Hillary Allen, another world-class trail runner who is now back to winning races after a life-threatening fall at the Tromsö Sky Race in 2017, who just happened to stop by. In just two days, five or six runners had just stopped in to say 'hi' before heading on their way and it struck me what an important central hub Barr Camp really is for the local running community.

It was a beautiful run down to town. There was barely a cloud in the sky and much of the snow had melted, leaving the trail clear and the views spectacular. What a magical experience. •

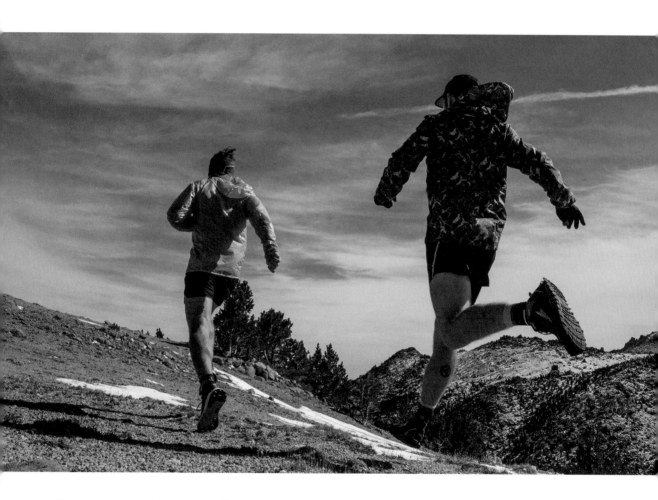

Race stats (selected)

2013 JFK 50-mile: 1st overall

2014 Lake Sonoma 50 Mile: 1st overall

2015 CCC Chamonix, France 101K: 1st overall (first American male to win any of the UTMB Series races)

2015 The North Face Endurance Challenge California 50-mile: 1st overall

2016 The North Face Endurance Challenge California 50-mile: 1st overall

2016 Madeira Island Ultra Trail Race, Portugal: 1st overall

CHAPTER FOUR

Desserts

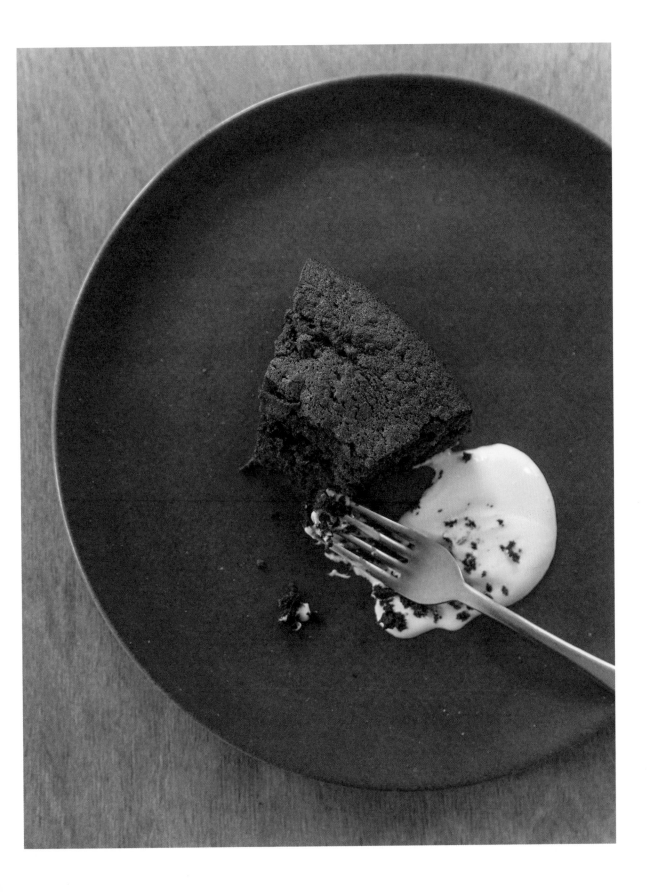

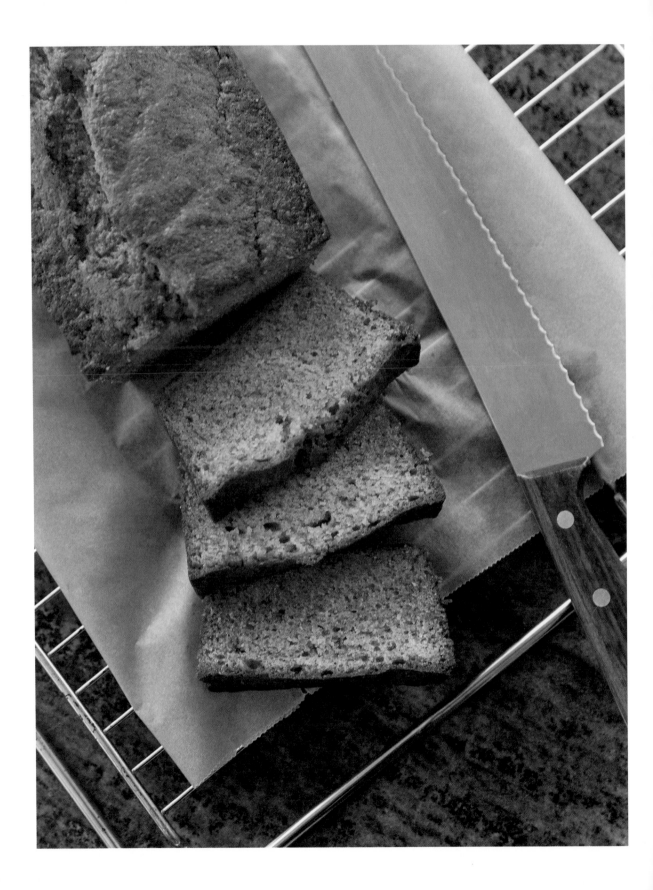

Ricky: 'I run to eat. Running allows me to eat what I want, without having to worry about whether I'm eating too much. I like cake and I probably do eat too much of it, but how much is too much? I do prefer to make my own cakes, as I know exactly what's gone into them. The trouble is, they're gone within a couple of days.'

RICKY LIGHTFOOT'S BANANA BREAD

SERVES 12

110g (4oz) butter, plus extra for greasing

225g (8oz) caster sugar

4 ripe bananas, mashed

85ml (generous $^1/_3$ cup) natural yogurt

2 free-range eggs, whisked

285g (10½oz) plain flour, sifted

1 tsp bicarbonate of soda

½ tsp salt

1. Preheat the oven to 180°C/350°F/Gas 4 and grease a 900g (2lb) loaf tin with a little butter.

2. In a large bowl, cream the butter and sugar together until fluffy and light. Add the mashed bananas, yogurt and whisked eggs and mix together, then fold in the flour, bicarbonate of soda and salt. Pour the batter into the prepared loaf tin.

3. Bake for 45–50 minutes, or until a skewer inserted into the cake comes out clean. If you can wait, turn out onto a wire rack and allow to cool before eating.

I love the flavour of rose in desserts – its subtle floral taste works great with strawberries. The dried petals add a bit of texture to this dish, but don't worry if you can't get hold of them.

STRAWBERRY AND ROSE RICE PUDDING

SERVES 4

200g (7oz) brown rice

1 litre (4 cups) milk (almond or oat milk work great for a vegan alternative)

3 tbsp honey or sugar

1 vanilla pod, split and seeds scraped out

300g (11oz) strawberries, washed, hulled and halved

5-6 drops rosewater

dried rose petals, to decorate (optional)

1. In a medium saucepan, combine the rice, milk, honey and vanilla and bring to a gentle simmer over a low heat. Gently simmer, stirring frequently, for 40–45 minutes until the rice is cooked and the mixture has thickened. If you find the mixture is getting too thick, you may need to add a little more milk from time to time. To test whether it's nearly ready, taste a few grains – they should be tender but with a little bit of bite remaining.

2. Fold one-third of the strawberries through the rice mixture along with the rosewater and simmer for a further 5 minutes.

3. Serve in dessert bowls, topped with the remaining strawberries and rose petals (if using).

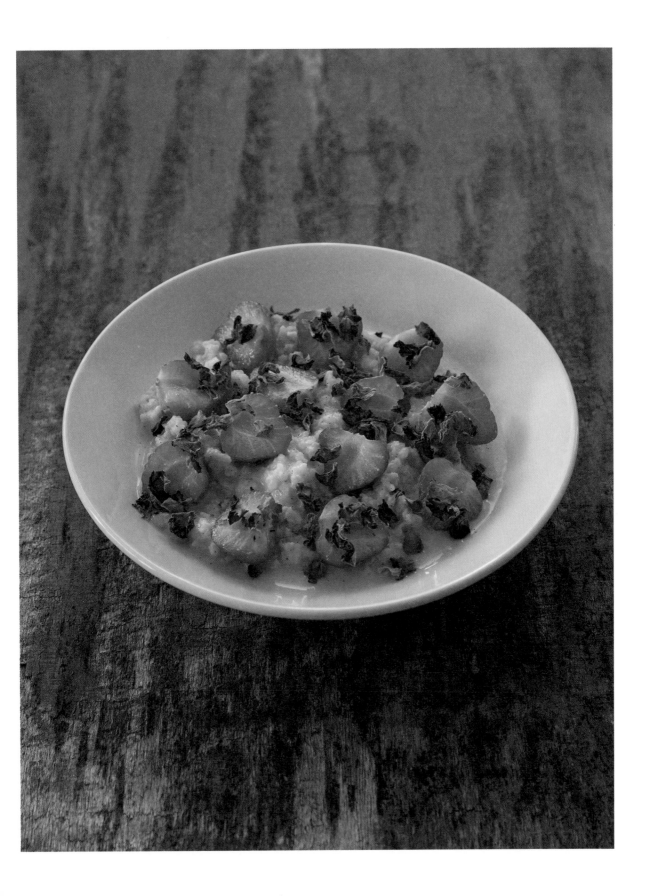

This is a quick dessert or a nice treat for yourself after a weekly long run –
I always have a version of this in the freezer. Greek yogurt is a great source
of protein and honey is a good sugar substitute. You can, of course, replace
the blueberries with any berry you like.

BLUEBERRY AND HONEY FROZEN YOGURT
WITH MINT AND FRESH BLUEBERRIES

SERVES 4

400g (14oz) full-fat Greek yogurt
150g (5oz) fresh or frozen blueberries
4 tbsp honey

TO SERVE:
150g (5oz) fresh blueberries
a few mint leaves, coarsely chopped

1. Put the ingredients into a bowl and mash them together with the back of a spoon until smooth (or lightly combine with a hand-held stick blender). Pour the mixture into a suitable freezerproof container and freeze for 4 hours, or until solid.

2. Remove from the freezer 10 minutes before serving, so that it softens a little. Enjoy sprinkled with fresh berries and some chopped mint.

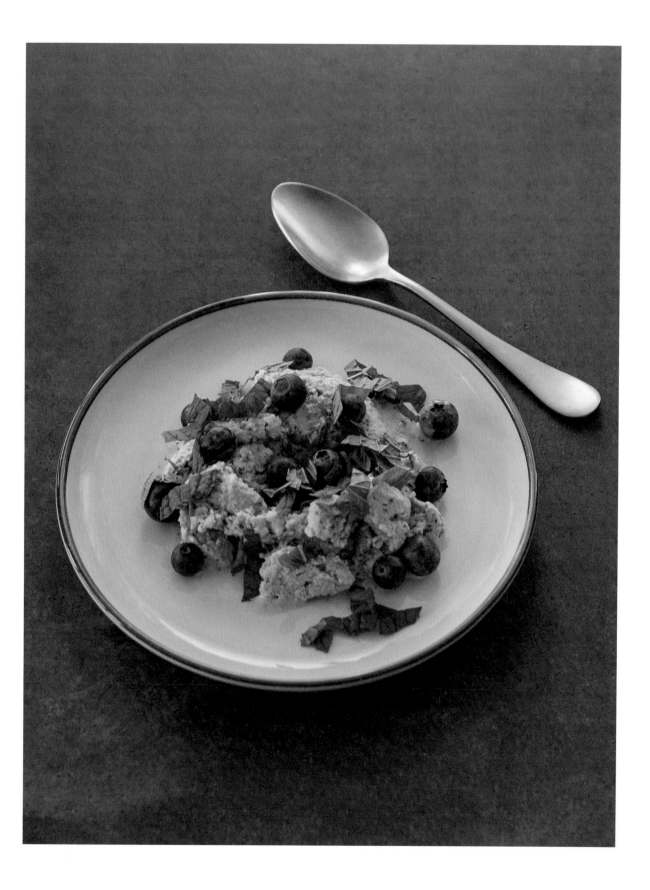

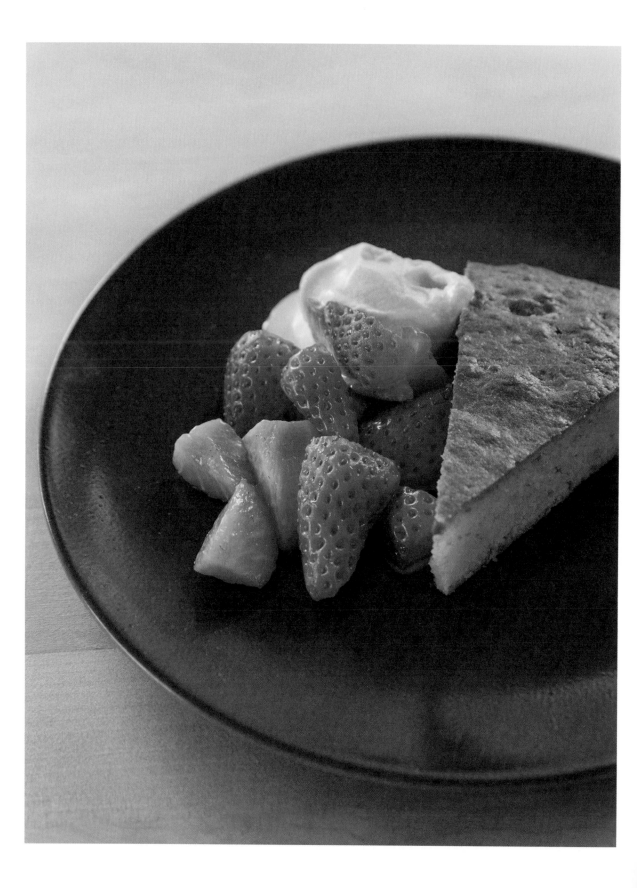

When Ricky Lightfoot told me of his cake obsession, I was happy; it gave me good reason to include this fragrant Greek-inspired cake in the book. Using olive oil brings a slightly bitter flavour, balanced out with the sweetness of the honey and the fresh lime zest. It is also much lower in saturated fat than butter.

The honey ice cream is the easiest ice cream recipe in the whole world and, because of the richness of the honey, you don't need to add egg yolks. It is not something for everyday, but it makes a lovely treat with none of the nasty additives you get in store-bought ice creams.

HONEY, YOGURT AND OLIVE OIL CAKE WITH HONEY ICE CREAM AND STRAWBERRIES

SERVES 8

FOR THE CAKE:
200ml (scant 1 cup) extra-virgin olive oil, plus extra for greasing
250g (9oz) full-fat Greek yogurt
200g (7oz) honey
finely grated zest of 1 lime
3 large (US extra large) eggs
250g (9oz) plain flour
½ tsp baking powder
½ tsp bicarbonate of soda
¼ tsp sea salt
fresh strawberries, to serve

FOR THE HONEY ICE CREAM:
200g (7oz) honey
750ml (3 cups) double or whipping cream

1. For the ice cream, lightly mix the honey and cream in a bowl or freezerproof container until well combined. Put it in the freezer, then mix every 15 minutes or so for 1½ hours until firm. If it gets too hard, bring it out of the freezer a few minutes before serving.

2. Preheat the oven to 180°C/350°F/Gas 4. Grease a 23cm (9in) round cake tin or springform pan with olive oil, line the base with baking paper, and grease the paper.

3. In a large bowl, whisk together the olive oil, yogurt, honey and lime zest. Add the eggs, one at a time, whisking well after each addition. Add the flour, baking powder, bicarbonate of soda and salt, and stir until the batter is almost smooth with just a few small lumps – don't overmix.

4. Transfer the batter to the tin and use a spatula to spread it evenly. Bake in the middle of the oven for 40–45 minutes until the top is lightly browned and an inserted skewer comes out clean. Let it cool in the tin for 10 minutes before turning out onto a wire rack (you may need to run a knife around the edge of the tin to loosen it).

5. Serve at room temperature with fresh strawberries and honey ice cream. Leftovers are nice the following day with a cup of tea, or packed up for a mid-run treat.

This is the most wonderful cake. The beetroot brings a moistness and a very slight earthy flavour that balances the bitterness of the chocolate and coffee. One of Mimmi Kotka's preferred pre-race treats is a big slice of chocolate cake – I'm certain she would approve of this one!

DARK CHOCOLATE AND BEETROOT CAKE

SERVES 8

200g (7oz) salted or unsalted butter (you choose), cut into small pieces, plus extra for greasing

250g (9oz) cooked and peeled beetroot

200g (7oz) dark chocolate (minimum 70 per cent cocoa solids), broken up

50ml (¼ cup) hot espresso or very strong black coffee

135g (4¾oz) plain flour

1 tsp baking powder

1 tsp bicarbonate of soda

3 tbsp unsweetened cocoa powder

5 free-range eggs, separated

190g (6½oz) golden caster sugar

crème fraîche, to serve

1. Preheat the oven to 180°C/350°F/Gas 4. Grease and line the base of a 20cm (8in) cake tin with baking paper.

2. Put the beetroot into a food processor and blend to a coarse purée. Set aside.

3. Melt the chocolate in a heatproof bowl suspended over a saucepan of hot water (don't allow the bottom of the bowl to touch the water), then pour in the hot coffee. Stir in the butter and let soften, then remove from the heat and cool slightly.

4. Meanwhile, sift together the flour, baking powder, bicarbonate of soda and cocoa in a large bowl and set aside.

5. Whisk the egg yolks in a bowl until frothy. Stir the egg yolks into the chocolate and butter mixture, then fold in the beetroot purée.

6. In a separate bowl, whisk the egg whites and slowly add the sugar until stiff peaks form. Fold into the chocolate mixture, then fold in the flour and cocoa mixture.

7. Pour the batter into the prepared tin and bake for 40–50 minutes, or until a skewer inserted into the cake comes out clean. Allow to cool in the tin before turning out. Serve with crème fraîche.

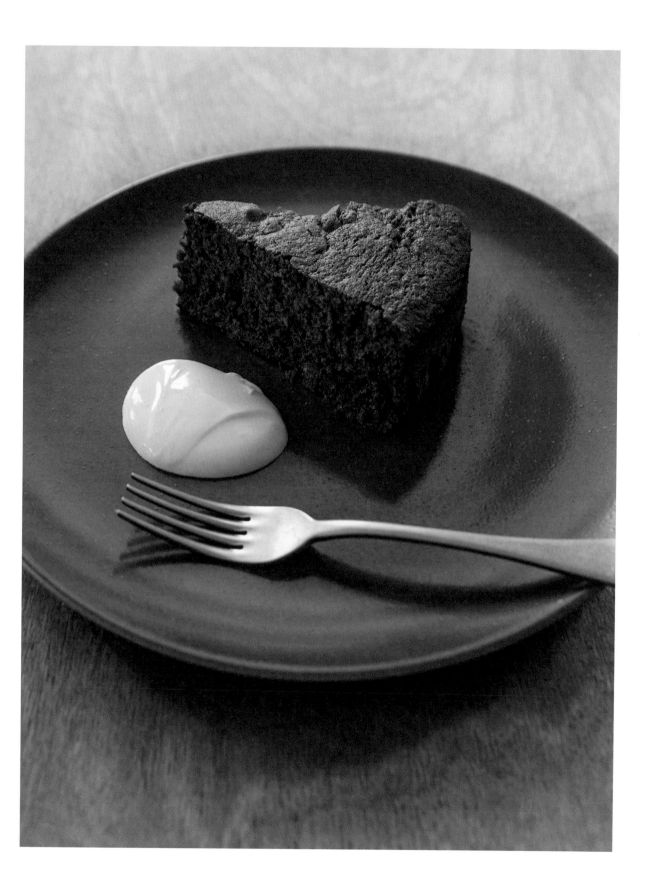

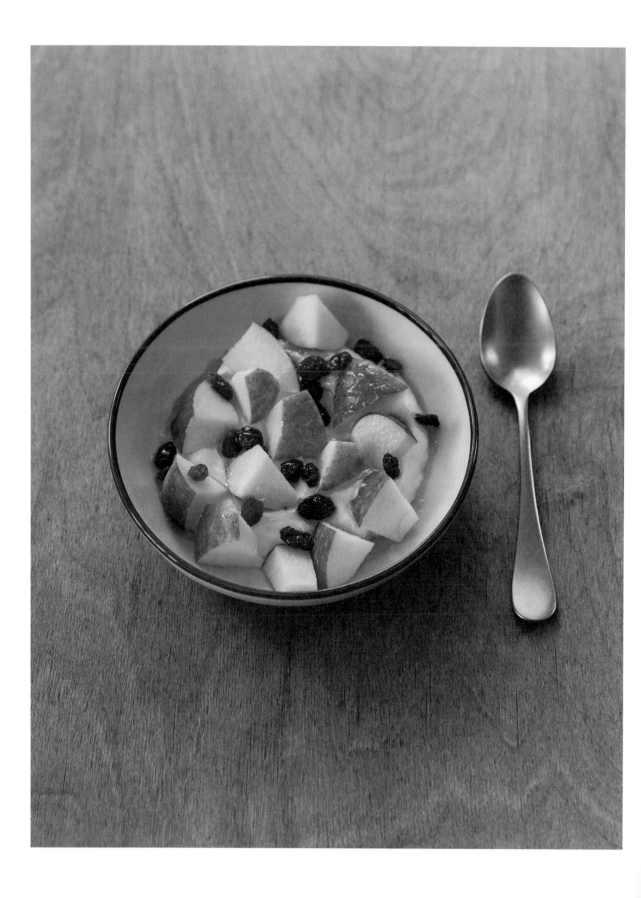

This isn't a recipe so much as a really quick and delicious thing to throw together after a run. It takes just a couple of minutes to prepare and gives you the calorie boost you need after exercising. The olive oil and salt give it a savoury touch, which I often crave. This is just one serving suggestion; you could also try chopped peaches and walnuts, or banana and hazlenuts.

GREEK YOGURT WITH APPLE, HONEY, OLIVE OIL AND SALT

SERVES 1

1 apple
4–5 tbsp Greek yogurt
1 tbsp raisins
honey, to taste
extra-virgin olive oil, to taste
a pinch of sea salt, to taste

1. Chop the apple into bite-size pieces (no need to peel, but discard the core).

2. Spoon the yogurt into a bowl, then top with the apple and raisins. Drizzle over a little honey and some olive oil and add a pinch of salt, to taste.

3. Eat immediately.

I didn't originally plan to make a dessert up at Barr Camp when I visited, but what better way to win the hearts of Zach Miller and the rest of the hikers than to make an apple crumble? Using dark sugar gives a deeper flavour and the touch of cinnamon brings a bit of an American feel!

APPLE CRUMBLE

SERVES 6

8 apples (Braeburn or Pink Lady), peeled, cored and chopped into large chunks

a handful of dark brown sugar

1 tbsp ground cinnamon

cream or Honey Ice Cream (see p.159), to serve

FOR THE TOPPING:

100g (3¾oz) wholemeal flour

100g (3¾oz) unsalted butter, diced into 1cm (²/₅in) pieces

50g (2oz) dark brown sugar

50g (2oz) rolled oats

1. Preheat the oven to 180°C/350°F/Gas 4.

2. In a large bowl, mix together the apples, sugar and cinnamon until evenly coated, then tumble the mixture into a deep baking tray or dish.

3. For the topping, in a separate bowl, gently rub the flour and butter together with your fingertips to a breadcrumb consistency, then add the sugar and oats and mix until well combined. Top the apples with the crumble topping mixture.

4. Bake for 30 minutes until the topping is evenly golden brown and a few spots of apple have started bubbling through.

5. Serve with cream or the Honey Ice Cream on p.159.

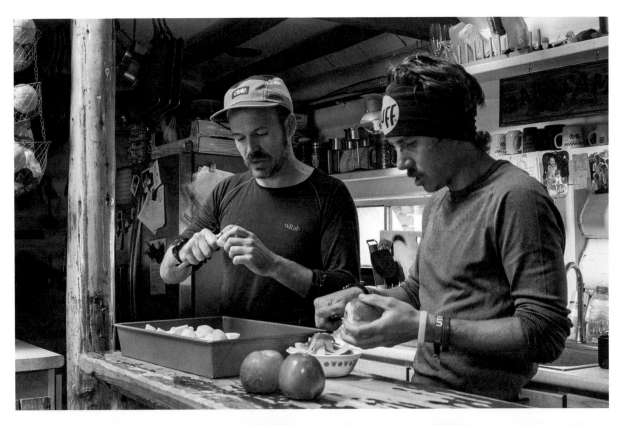

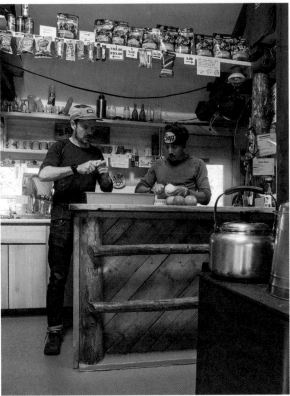

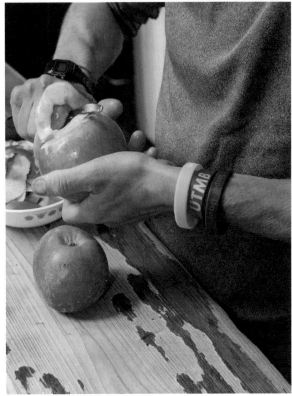

On the Trail with:

Emelie Forsberg, Ida Nilsson and Mimmi Kotka

Sweden

ON A MISTY autumn morning in the archipelago just outside Stockholm, I lit a small fire ready to cook some breakfast for three of the world's best mountain runners: Ida Nilsson, Mimmi Kotka and Emelie Forsberg; three women who are not only world-class athletes but who also just set up their own organic sports nutrition brand, Moonvalley.

Before we ate, we shared a small run in the forest and over the treacherously slippery rocks. The sun was breaking through the mist and it promised to be a beautiful day. When we got back, I cooked up cep and chanterelle mushrooms with just a little garlic and olive oil; grilled some tomatoes; made

Rainbow Chard, Squash and Brown Rice Tortilla (see p.58); and finally served up some Rye and Oat Porridge (see p. 23).

We sat around the fire to eat and talk about food – a favourite subject – and the energy that they brought with them was infectious. I loved listening to them talk about everything, from childhood tastes to mushroom picking. Self-confessed foodies, all three have a background in food: Ida trained as a chef and has worked in private ski chalets and restaurants in the French Alps; Emelie is an experienced baker and lives on her own small sustainable farm in northern Norway;

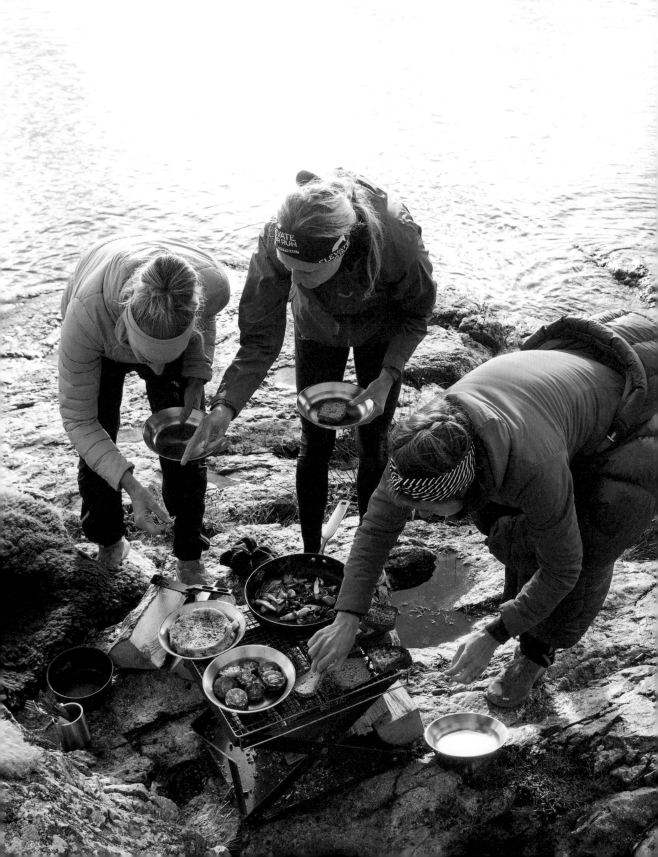

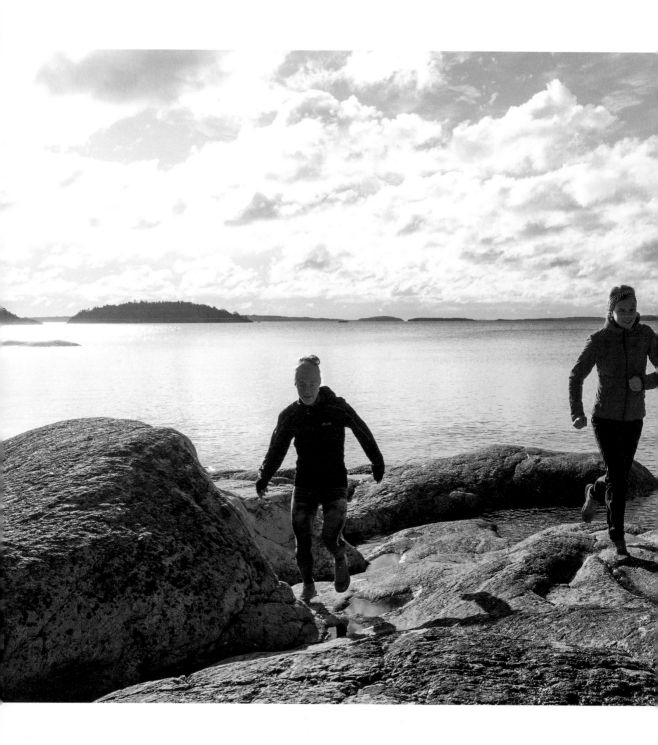

EMELIE • IDA • MIMMI

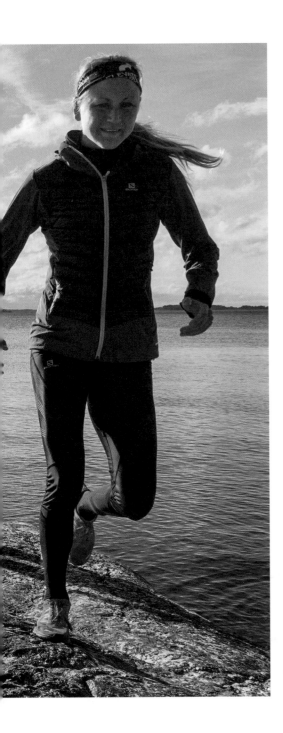

and Mimmi has a master's degree in food science and molecular nutrition. What better people to talk to about eating for endurance running?

We talked about how to fuel yourself in the best possible way, without leaving yourself depleted, after training and racing – both activities that have huge effects on the body. Mimmi, reflecting her background in food science, pointed out that there are some potentially dangerous side effects from following very low-carb diets in the long term, especially for female endurance runners. Around 60 per cent of female endurance athletes are undernourished, with calorie deficiency and a lack of iron in particular in their diets.

When it comes to eating to sustain endurance running, it's an absolute must to eat plenty of food, that contains a varied selection of protein, carbohydrates and fats, with as little industrially processed produce as possible.

Only Emelie is a strict vegetarian, but both Mimmi and Ida pay attention to the amount of meat they eat, focusing on more plant-based proteins such as beans and pulses than animal products. When it comes to carbs, they all steer away from 'white' carbs in favour of whole grains and root vegetables. And in terms of fats, they believe that unrefined oils such as olive oil and coconut oil are great, but that you shouldn't be afraid of a little

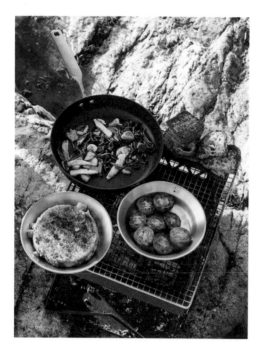

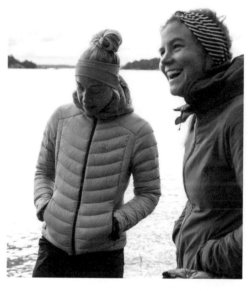

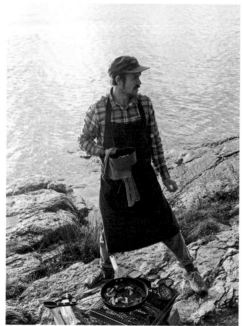

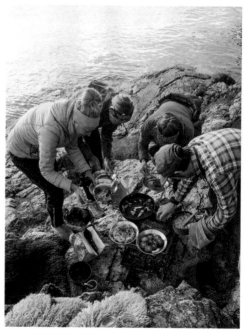

EMELIE • IDA • MIMMI

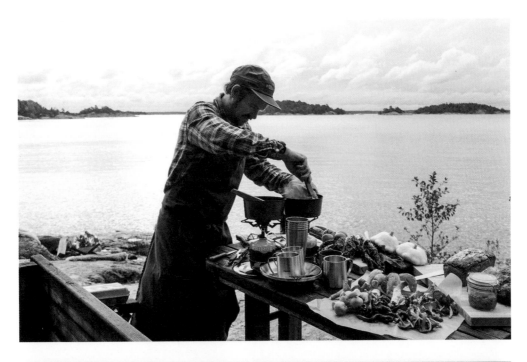

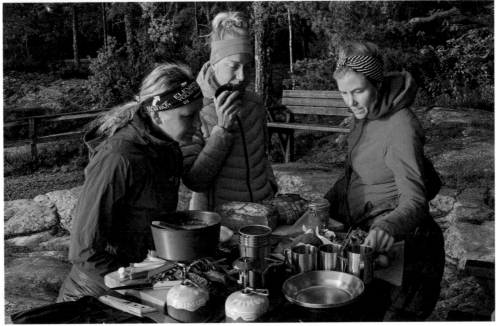

EMELIE • IDA • MIMMI

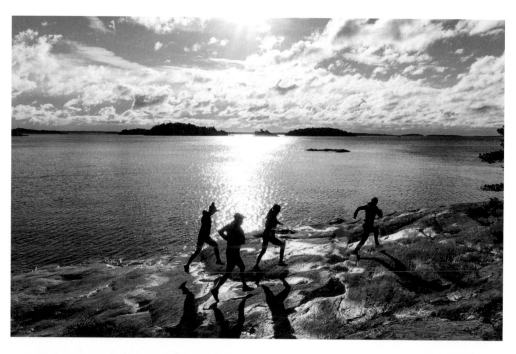

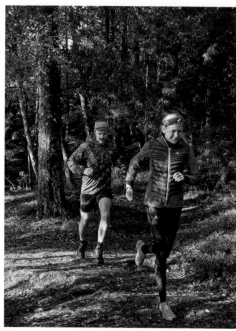

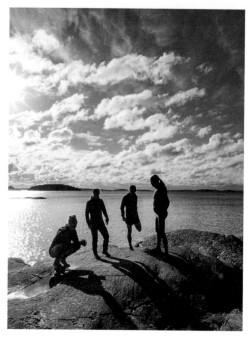

EMELIE • IDA • MIMMI

«Just as there is no single workout that will make you a good runner, there is no single food that you eat before a race that will make you perform better. It's what you are eating in your day-to-day life that matters.»

_____

butter. Another thing that really came across loud and clear was that having the odd treat is essential – cinnamon buns were mentioned on more than one occasion!

We also talked about the environmental impact of our diets, a subject that the three of them care about greatly. Emelie reflected: 'If you are interested in nature and visiting these beautiful places, how can you not be interested in what you eat, especially when your diet can have such major negative effects on the environment?'

Ida agreed, 'For me, food is closely linked to living in harmony with the local environment. I like to pick things in the forest, planting and growing myself, or buying local produce. I find this more interesting and fun to focus on than sports nutrition. Of course, I want to fuel my body for training and performance as well, but it's more enjoyable to think about the food that comes from where I live or where I'm staying at that moment. It's a way to get my body in sync with that place.

'I don't have a standard pre- or post-run meal. Just as there is no single workout that will make you a good runner, there is no single food that you eat before a race that will make you perform

better. It's what you are eating in your day-to-day life that matters. I usually eat what I can get depending on the season or where in the world it is I'm running.'

We share very similar thoughts when it comes to the food we eat. Their advice for eating was sensible, whether you are a runner or not: learn to cook; eat local; eat good unprocessed carbs; follow a Nordic or Mediteranean diet that is high in whole grains and fresh produce; and don't over-complicate things – if you are making a spaghetti bolognese, just add extra veggies to get more nutrients.

Likewise, their training methods were all very intuitive. They work with some structured speed, some hill work and long runs, but mainly listen to what their bodies tell them and don't overdo it. One thing that all three stressed was how important rest is. Mimmi even said she would rather go into a race 10 per cent undertrained than 1 per cent over-trained. In fact, Mimmi summed up the philosophy of all three best when she said 'to perform well and have the longevity you desire in this sport, you must be well-fed, well-rested and happy'. •

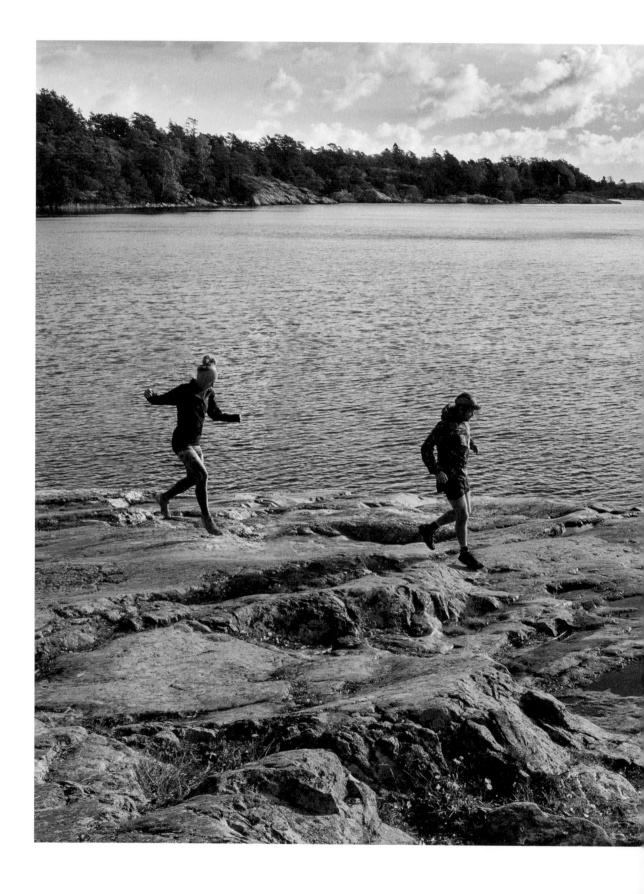

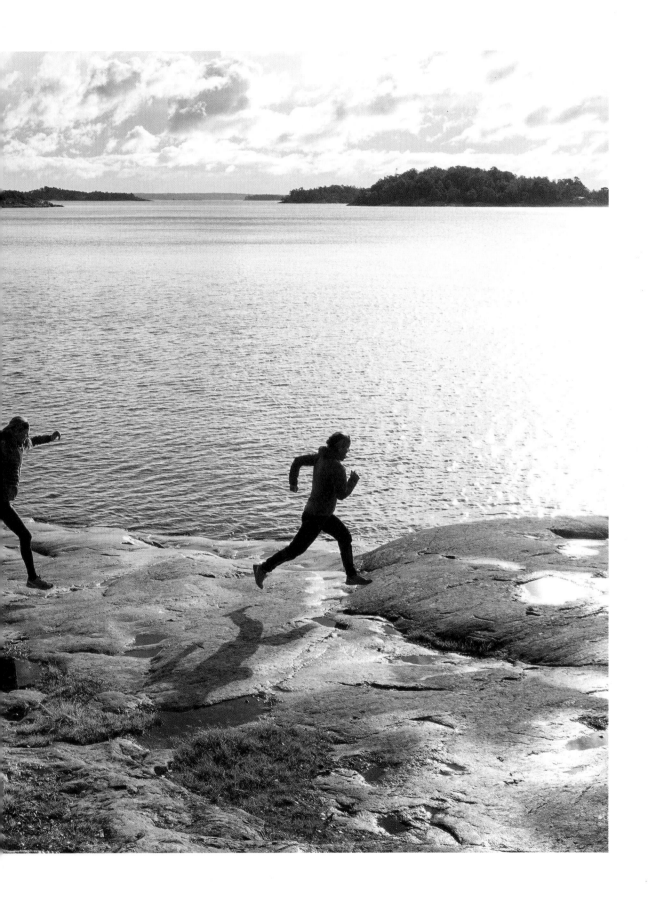

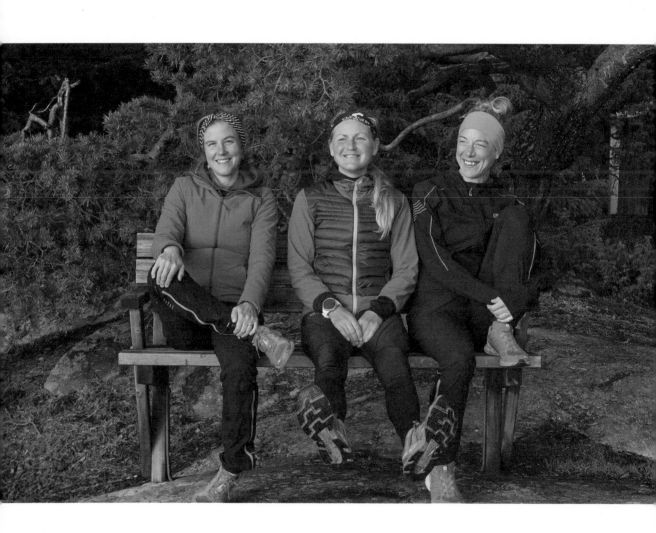

EMELIE • IDA • MIMMI

Race stats (selected)

Emelie Forsberg

2014 Skyrunning world champion
2015 Skyrunning world cup winner
2017 Glen Coe Skyline: winner and course record
2018 Kungsleden: FKT (fastest known time)
Mont Blanc: FKT
Matterhorn: FKT
Kebnekaise: FKT

Mimmi Kotka

2016 CCC: winner
2017 TDS: course record
2018 Mont Blanc 90K: course record

Ida Nilsson

2016, 2017, 2018 Transvulcania Ultra Marathon: winner
2016, 2017 The North Face Endurance Challenge 50-miles: 1st female
2017 Ultravasan 90K: winner
2018 Zegama Marathon: winner

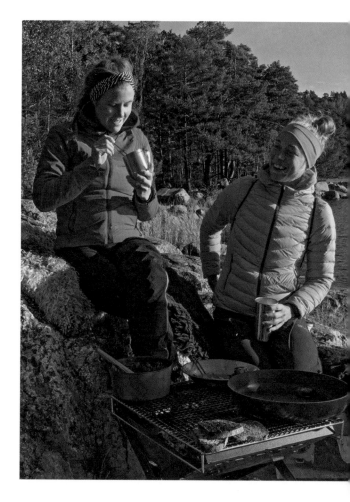

CHAPTER FIVE

Storecupboard Staples

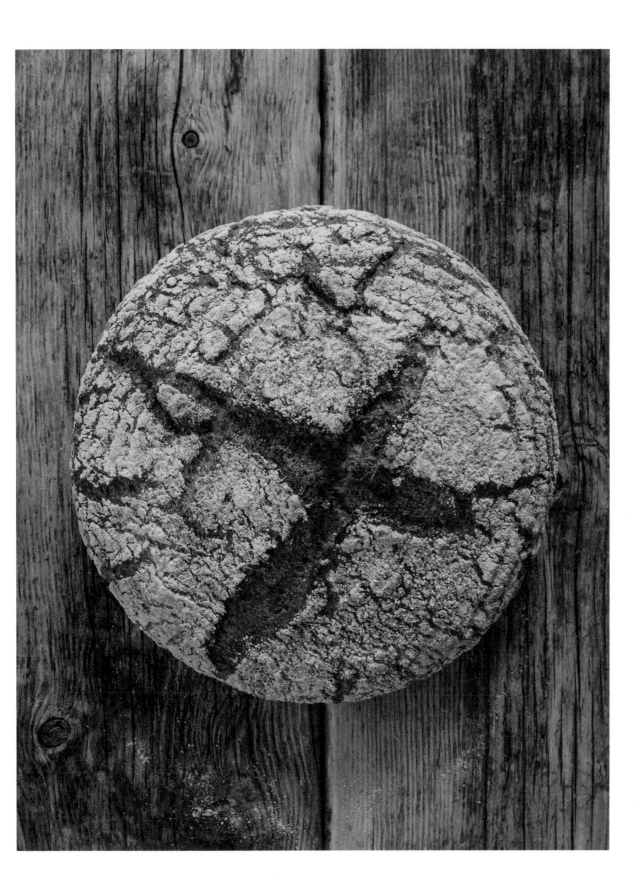

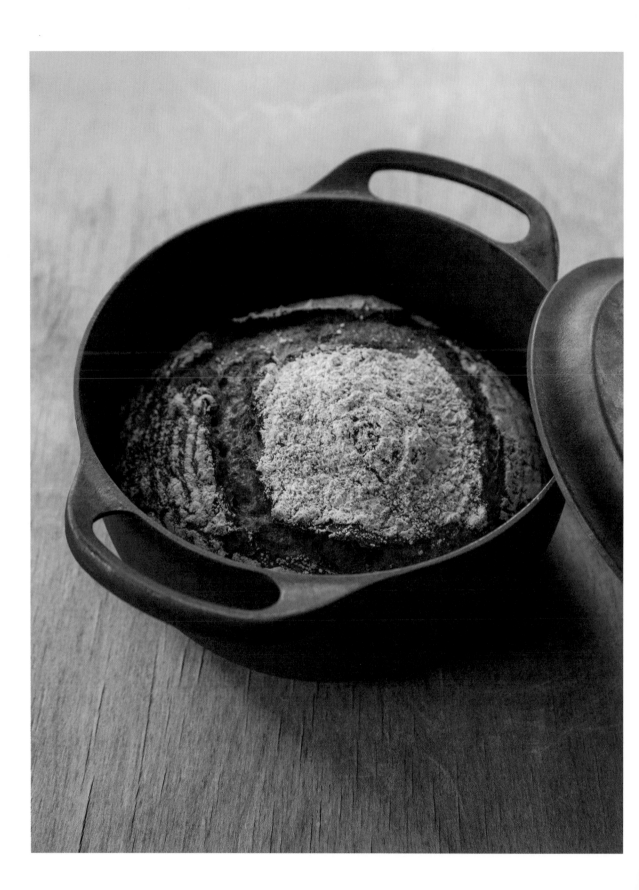

Bread

Bread is often villified as something we shouldn't eat or that is bad for us, but in my opinion a sourdough bread that is home-baked or bought from a good bakery, with whole grains and with no (or minimal) additives other than flour, water and salt, is a good source of wholegrain carbohydrates and so much better than mushy white sliced or overly sweet malty breads from the supermarket. A longer process of fermentation breaks down the gluten and phytic acid molecules, which makes the bread much more digestible and releases a lot more of the nutrients available in the grains.

Always use the best flour you can get hold of; organic grains sourced from a small mill will have such a positive effect on the flavour of the bread you bake, that once you have tried it, it will be impossible for you to go back to standard flour.

Baking with a 100 per cent sourdough starter is a bit of a tricky process. As far as I've learned, it's not so much of an exact science. It depends on various things: heat, humidity and the strength or weakness of the flours used.

To begin, you need a sourdough starter, also known as a 'Mother'. I started my Mother about seven years ago. It's a simple process of mixing flour and water, which you then leave at room temperature for a few days for the wild yeasts and bacteria to get going.

A piece of baking equipment I find essential is a Swedish 1dl (100ml)/scant ½ cup volume measuring cup – it saves weighing all the ingredients, making the process far less laborious. For those who don't have a dl measuring cup, I have also given the amounts in US cups and in grams.

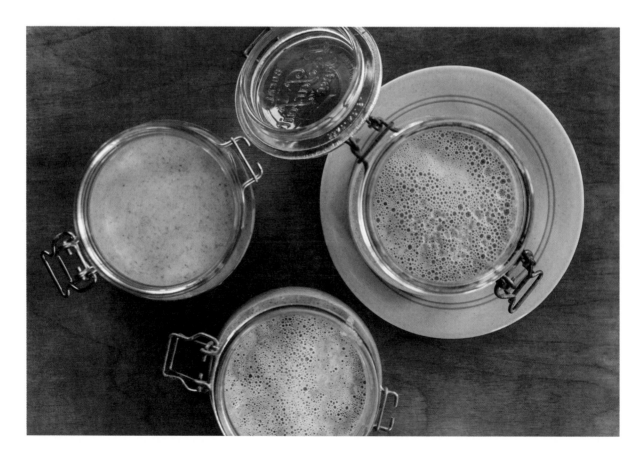

SOURDOUGH STARTER ('THE MOTHER')

MAKES 1½ CUPS (420G/3DL)

1kg (2¼lb) wholewheat flour
1kg (2¼lb) strong bread flour
water

Note: The conversions are not
interchangeable, so don't mix
measurements – stick to one system.

DAY 1

Mix the flours together and store in an
airtight container – keep this 50/50 flour
mix to hand, to feed the starter.

In a ceramic bowl, mix 1 cup (120g/2dl)
of 50/50 flour mix with 1 cup (200ml/2dl)
water to make a thick paste. Loosely cover
with a clean tea towel and leave at room
temperature for 24 hours.

DAY 2

The following day, feed the mixture with ½
cup (60g/1dl) of 50/50 flour mix and ½ cup
(100ml/1dl) water. Mix together – if there is
a skin on the top, mix that in too. Re-cover
and leave at room temperature.

DAY 3

You may begin to see signs of life at this
point and there may be a few bubbles on
the top of the mixture. Repeat the Day 2
process.

DAY 4

You will almost certainly see signs of
fermentation. Repeat the Day 2 process.

DAY 5

By now, it should be smelling tangy and full
of bubbles. Remove ½ cup (140g/1dl) of the
Mother to a clean ceramic bowl and repeat
the Day 2 process. Discard the leftover. This
will feel wasteful, but it's a small price to
pay for a lifetime of sourdough baking.

DAY 6

Repeat the entire Day 5 process.

DAY 7

The Mother is ready to bake with!

You can re-feed your Mother after
breadmaking and bake more the following
day. Alternatively, you can store it in the
refrigerator, but it will need to be fed as
from Day 5 to get it back up and running
again. It will keep in the refrigerator for
many months before it needs to be re-fed. It
will develop a layer of brown liquid on the
top after a couple of weeks – this is a kind of
wild vinegar and is nothing to worry about:
just pour it off and mix the hibernating
Mother with fresh flour and water to restart.

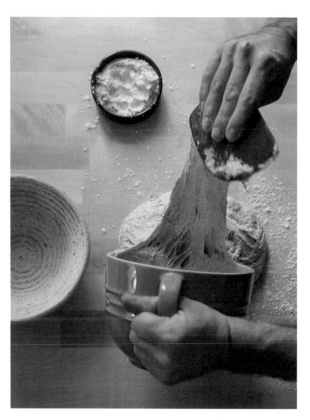
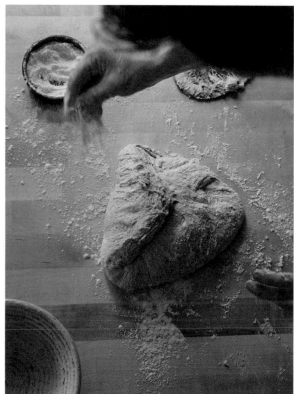
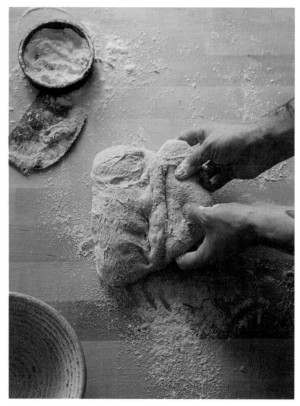
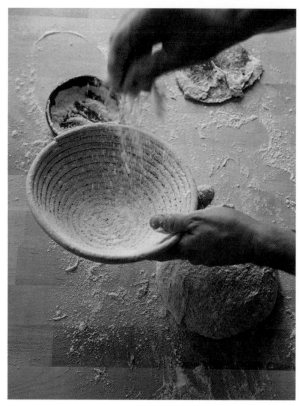

I always recommend getting started with this loaf. Once you get the feel of baking with sourdough, then the experiments can begin! At home, I bake in a cast-iron pot, like an old-fashioned Dutch oven. Baking with the lid on for the first half of baking steams the bread, then removing the lid for the last half gives the most amazing crust. Alternatively, use a baking tray and place a shallow saucepan of water on the shelf below to create some steam.

BASIC SOURDOUGH BREAD

MAKES 1 LOAF

2 cups (240g/4dl) strong white flour
1 cup (120g/2dl) wholegrain flour
1 cup (280g/2dl) Sourdough Starter/ Mother (see p.183)
2 cups (400ml/4dl) water
2 tsp (10g/²/₅oz) salt

Note: The conversions are not interchangeable, so don't mix measurements – stick to one system.

1. Put the flours, sourdough starter and water into a stand mixer fitted with a dough hook attachment and mix slowly for 2–3 minutes until a sticky dough is formed. Cover with a clean tea towel and allow to rest for 20 minutes.

2. Add the salt to the dough and mix on medium speed for a further 6–8 minutes until the dough looks smooth and is slightly springy to the touch.

3. Transfer the dough to a clean ceramic bowl, cover with a tea towel and allow to prove for 2–3 hours in a warm place until almost doubled in size. You can leave the dough overnight in the refrigerator, if you prefer. This will slow down the fermentation, but also give the finished bread a sourer flavour.

4. Use a dough scraper or silicone spatula to turn the dough onto a lightly floured work surface and allow to rest for 15 minutes. Flatten the dough slightly, then bring the 4 opposite sides of the dough into the centre, one at a time. Flip the dough over so the seam is on the bottom and shape into a tight ball. Either place the ball of dough into a well-floured dough basket or leave it on a wooden board, well dusted with flour and covered with a tea towel. Leave in a warm place for 1–2 hours until plump and very springy to the touch.

5. Preheat the oven to 250°C/500°F/Gas 10 and put the cast-iron pot in the oven to heat up.

6. Carefully put the risen dough into the cast-iron pot (with the patterned side facing up, if you have used a dough basket) and score the top with a razor blade or a very sharp knife. Put the lid on the pot and bake for 20 minutes, then remove the lid, reduce the oven temperature to 220°C/425°F/Gas 7 and bake for a further 20 minutes. Carefully take the bread out of the pot and tap the bottom – it should sound hollow and feel light. If not, bake for a further 5 minutes.

7. Leave the bread to cool on a wire rack. I challenge you to not have a slice!

Polenta is gluten free, so makes an easy-to-digest loaf, although my main reason to make this is for the taste: the slight sweetness of the polenta and subtle aniseed flavour of the fennel seeds is a real treat. Lightly toasted and rubbed with a raw garlic clove it makes a great bruschetta.

POLENTA, FENNEL AND SESAME BREAD

MAKES 1 LOAF

1½ cups (200g/3dl) polenta flour

1½ cups (180g/3dl) strong white bread flour

1 cup (280g/2dl) Sourdough Starter/Mother (see p.183)

2 cups (400ml/4dl) water

½ cup (60g/1dl) sesame seeds

3 tbsp fennel seeds

2½ tsp (12g/2½oz) salt

Note: The conversions are not interchangeable, so don't mix measurements - stick to one system.

1. Put the flours, sourdough starter and water into a stand mixer fitted with a dough hook attachment and mix slowly for 2–3 minutes until a sticky dough is formed.

2. Mix the seeds together in a separate bowl. Reserve 2 tablespoons of seeds for topping, then add the remaining seeds to the dough and mix slowly until the seeds are evenly incorporated. Cover with a clean tea towel and allow to rest for 20 minutes.

3. Add the salt to the dough and mix on medium speed for a further 6–8 minutes.

4. Prove and bake, following the same method as the recipe for Basic Sourdough Bread (see p.185). Before scoring, brush the top of the loaf with a little water and top with the reserved seeds.

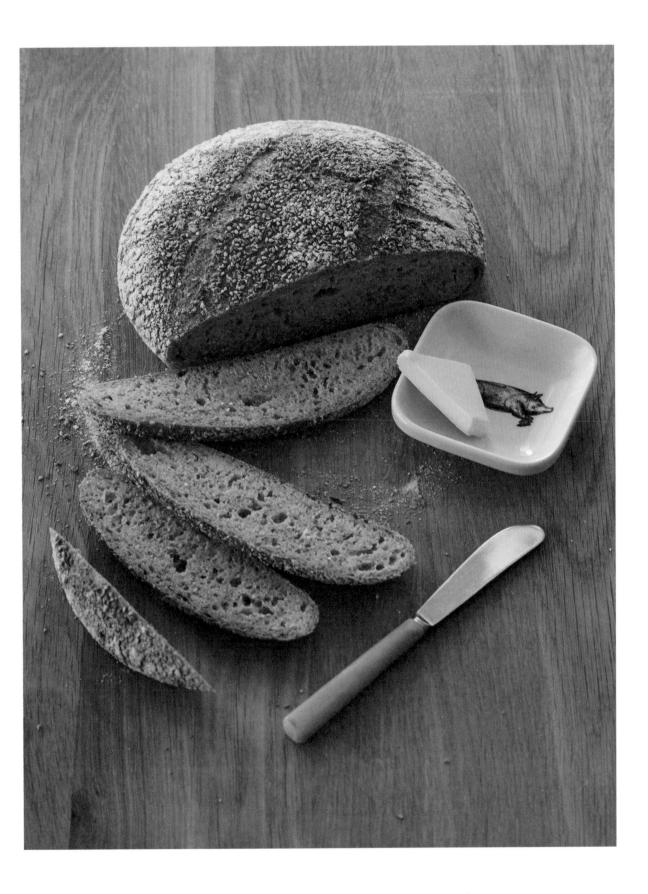

Rye bread is much denser than the other breads here, but the flavour is sweeter than that of wheat and rye has a much lower gluten content, which can make it easier to digest when out for a run. This is especially good spread with the Walnut and Date Butter on p.199.

RYE AND WALNUT LOAF

MAKES 1 LOAF

1 cup (120g/2dl) wholegrain rye flour

2 cups (240g/4dl) strong white bread flour

1 cup (280g/2dl) Sourdough Starter/ Mother (see p.183)

2½ cups (500ml/5dl) water

½ cup (50g/1dl) chopped toasted walnuts

2 tsp (10g/²/₅oz) salt

Note: The conversions are not interchangeable, so don't mix measurements – stick to one system.

1. Put the flours, sourdough starter and water into a stand mixer fitted with a dough hook attachment and mix slowly for 2–3 minutes until a sticky dough is formed.

2. Add the walnuts to the dough and mix slowly until the nuts are evenly incorporated. The dough will look quite loose – this is okay, as the rye flour will soak up the extra liquid during the resting period. Cover with a clean tea towel and allow to rest for 20 minutes.

3. Add the salt to the dough and mix on medium speed for a further 6–8 minutes.

4. Prove and bake, following the same method as the recipe for Basic Sourdough Bread (see p.185), but add an extra 5 minutes to the baking time.

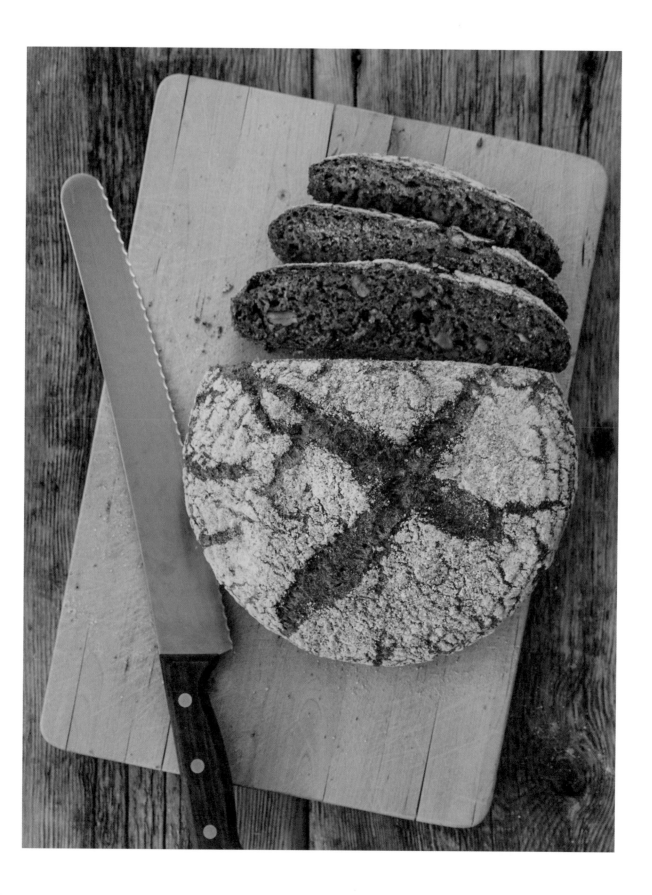

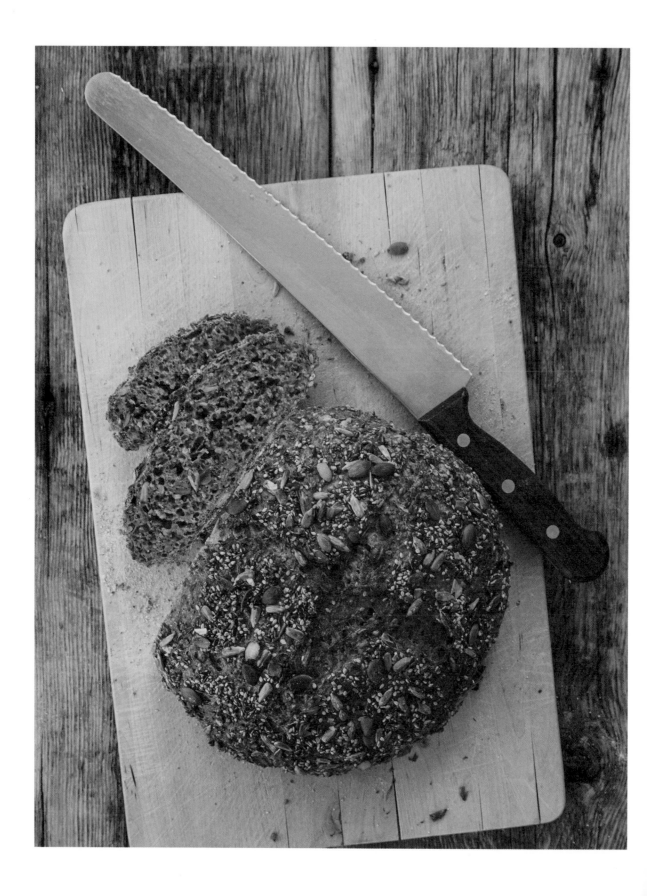

This variation on the basic sourdough loaf is great for runners. When it comes to the health benefits of quinoa, the list is almost endless, the spelt flour has a higher protein content than wheat flour and the seeds are also very nutrient-rich. This bread is slightly denser in texture than the basic sourdough due to the added extras.

I highly recommend this spread with one of the nut butters on p.199, especially for taking out on a long run. It takes some practice to walk briskly up a hill eating a nut butter sandwich, but it's worth it for the energy boost.

SEEDED QUINOA LOAF

MAKES 1 LOAF

2 cups (240g/4dl) strong white bread flour

½ cup (60g/1dl) wholegrain spelt flour (or you can use wholegrain wheat or einkorn)

½ cup (80g/1dl) quinoa

1 cup (280g/2dl) Sourdough Starter/ Mother (see p.183)

2¼ cups (450ml/4½dl) water

2 tbsp chia seeds

2 tbsp flax seeds

2 tbsp sesame seeds

4 tbsp pumpkin seeds

4 tbsp sunflower seeds

2½ tsp (12g/2½oz) salt

Note: The conversions are not interchangeable, so don't mix measurements - stick to one system.

1. Put the flours, quinoa, sourdough starter and water into a stand mixer fitted with a dough hook attachment and mix slowly for 2–3 minutes until a sticky dough is formed.

2. Mix all the seeds together in a separate bowl. Reserve 2 tablespoons of seeds for topping, then add the remaining seeds to the dough and mix slowly until the seeds are evenly incorporated. The dough will look quite loose – this is okay, as the chia and flax seeds will soak up the extra liquid during the resting period. Cover with a clean tea towel and allow to rest for 20 minutes.

3. Add the salt to the dough and mix on medium speed for a further 6–8 minutes.

4. Prove and bake, following the same method as the recipe for Basic Sourdough Bread (see p.185). Before scoring, brush the top of the loaf with a little water and top with the reserved seeds.

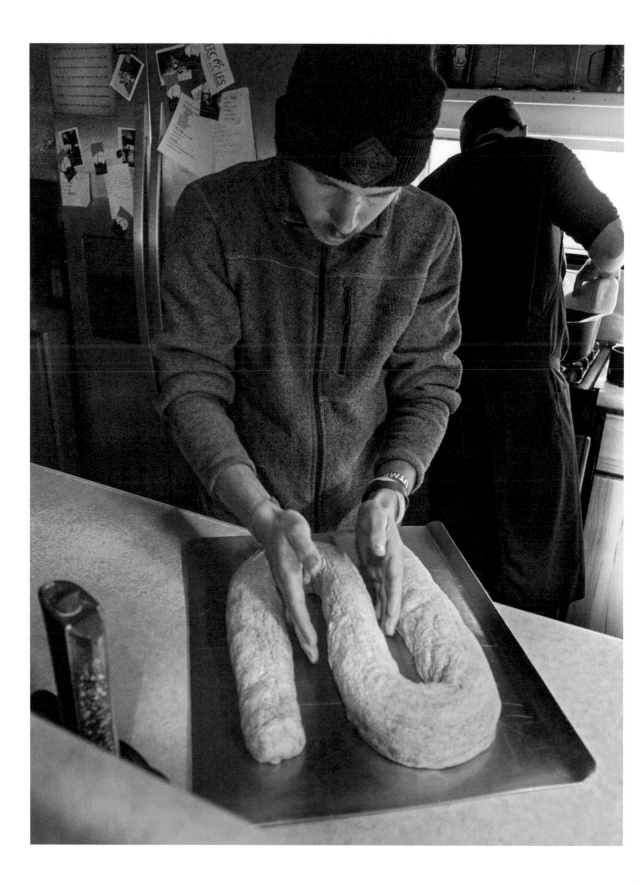

Hundreds of hikers and runners are met every year at Barr Camp with the delicious smell of freshly baked garlic bread – a welcome aroma, marking that you are almost at your destination, after at least two hours of hiking from Manitou Springs up the Barr trail. It's a staple on the menu and for very good reason – who doesn't love garlic bread?! A versatile recipe, it's also good topped with chopped nuts and brown sugar.

BARR CAMP SWITCHBACK GARLIC BREAD

SERVES 5-6

vegetable oil, for greasing
milk, for brushing (at Barr Camp they use evaporated milk)
sea salt, to taste
dried minced garlic, to taste

FOR THE DOUGH:
235ml (scant 1 cup) warm water
1 tbsp active dried yeast
2 tbsp sugar (any type)
¼ tsp salt
170g (6oz) plain flour
130g (4½oz) wholewheat flour
100g (3¾oz) buckwheat flour

1. In a large bowl, mix together the water, yeast, sugar and salt. Add the flours, one at a time, mixing well after each addition, until you have a dough that is easy to handle (not sticky and not tough). Knead until smooth, then place back in the bowl and set aside to rise in a warm place for 1 hour, or until at least doubled in size.

2. Meanwhile, preheat the oven to 180°C/350°F/ Gas 4 and grease a large baking tray with vegetable oil.

3. Roll out the dough on the work surface into a long 'rope', about 45–60cm (18–24in) long. Place the dough on the baking tray, curling it into whatever shape you like: a zig-zag, circle, heart, horseshoe, whatever. Brush the dough all over with milk, then sprinkle with salt and dried garlic to taste.

4. Bake for 40 minutes, or until crisp and well browned. Enjoy!

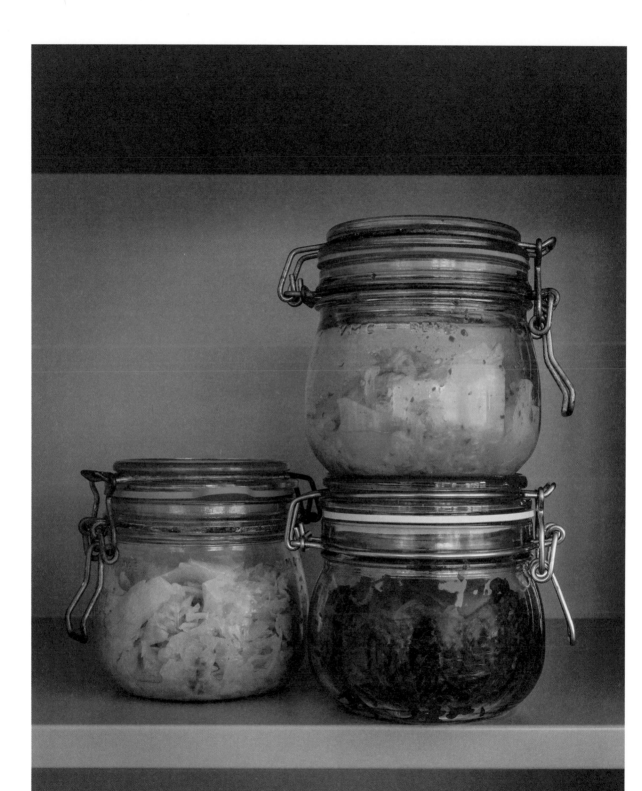

Fermentation

Fermentation is something we comfortably live with in our daily lives; bread, cheese, yogurt, wine and beer would all be absent from your refrigerator and cupboards without it. However, when it comes to fermenting vegetables at home without refrigeration (a process known as lacto-fermentation) we tend to get a little nervous – I was the first time I tried it! Lacto-fermenting vegetables is not a dangerous method of preservation. Apart from the safety of knowing that the salt will destroy potentially harmful bacteria, if the product has begun to rot rather than ferment it will be immediately apparent, as it will be completely unappetising.

Lacto-fermenting vegetables is something that almost every culture the world over has been doing for thousands of years. Before refrigeration, this was a way to preserve the bounty of the summer's harvest. More recently, people have been looking into the health benefits of these foods. In Korea and Japan, heavily salted fermented fruits are served after meals to aid digestion; yogurt bacteria is known to help improve the digestion of lactose; and the longer process of baking with a sourdough starter rather than conventional yeast can help to break down the starches that can cause some gluten-related inflammatory gut issues. The health properties of fermented foods are clear and, as interest in the microbiome and gut flora is growing, I think these 'living foods' will become a bigger part of our diets.

Most important for me is the flavour and depth that fermented vegetables can bring to your cooking – they are delicious! The flavour of fermented foods can often be an acquired taste, but these two simple recipes will effectively start you off at the beginning and will become welcome additions to your larder. Start off by trying some store-bought sauerkraut and kimchi, so that you have a reference point of what you should be aiming for. Remember, though, the homemade version will always be much better than store-bought!

KIMCHI

1kg (2¼lb) Chinese cabbage, chopped into 3cm (1¼in) pieces

200g (7oz) spring onions (scallions), finely sliced

200g (7oz) daikon radish, finely sliced

3 red chillies

a thumb-sized piece of fresh root ginger

60g (2⅓oz) garlic cloves, peeled

25g (1oz) sea salt

1. Combine the cabbage, spring onions and radish in a spotlessly clean mixing bowl.

2. Put the chillies, ginger, garlic and salt into a food processor and process to a paste.

3. With clean hands, work the paste into the chopped vegetables, kneading to get as much liquid out of the vegetables as possible. Pack the mixture into a sterilised glass jar and and pour over the liquid. Press firmly down on the veg to make sure there are no air bubbles and that they are fully submerged, and weight the contents down (a handful of baking beans tied securely into a double freezer bag works well). Cover the jar loosely with the lid, to allow the fermenting gasses to escape.

4. Set it in a dark, slightly warm place for 1–2 days, then check on it to make sure it has begun to ferment – there should be small, rising bubbles visible. If so, it can be moved to a slightly cooler place – no warmer than room temperature. The cooler the temperature, the longer it will take to be ready. After another 3 days, and when the bubbling has subsided, taste it. It should taste sour and the longer you leave it fermenting, the sourer it will get. Keep tasting it until you are happy with the flavour, then remove the weight, place the lid on tightly and refrigerate. It will keep for at least 1 month in the refrigerator.

This traditional sauerkraut can happily be flavoured with any number of additions, such as juniper berries and caraway seeds, grated apple or beets, horseradish or fresh dill. Simply add them to the jar when bottling.

RED SAUERKRAUT

MAKES 1 X 1-LITRE (4-CUP) JAR

1kg (2¼lb) red cabbage
20g (¾oz) sea salt

Note: To make Fennel Sauerkraut, simply follow the recipe above, but replace the cabbage with the same weight of fennel. This method also works well with white cabbage.

1. Wash the cabbage and slice it very finely (a food processor or mandoline is helpful for this). Place it in a spotlessly clean mixing bowl along with the sea salt and massage with clean hands to mix well. Allow to stand for at least 15 minutes.

2. With clean hands, knead and squeeze the cabbage, trying to get as much liquid out of it as possible. Pack the cabbage into a sterilised glass jar and pour over the liquid. Press firmly down on the cabbage to make sure there are no air bubbles and that the cabbage is fully submerged. Weight the contents down (a handful of baking beans tied securely into a double freezer bag works well) and cover the jar loosely with the lid, to allow the fermenting gasses to escape.

3. Set it in a dark, slightly warm place for 1–2 days, then check on it to make sure it has begun to ferment – there should be small, rising bubbles visible. If so, it can be moved to a slightly cooler place – no warmer than room temperature. The cooler the temperature, the longer it will take to be ready. After another 3 days, and when the bubbling has subsided, taste it. It should taste sour and the longer you leave it fermenting, the sourer it will get. Keep tasting it until you are happy with the flavour, then remove the weight, place the lid on tightly and refrigerate. It will keep for at least 1 month in the refrigerator.

Nut Butters

Everyone is familiar with peanut butter, but homemade nut butters using other nut varieties have a higher nutritional value and are also in a different league when it comes to taste. They take next to no time to make, and there are no added sugars or nasty preservatives. With healthy fats, plenty of protein and slow-burning carbohydrates, nuts are a great addition to a runner's diet.

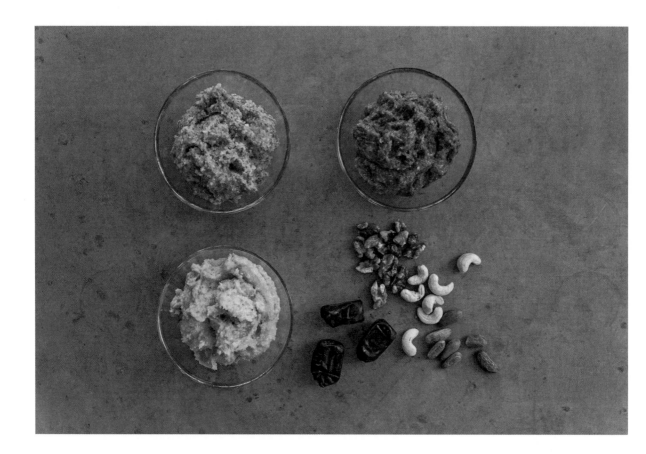

This butter is quite mild in taste, so it's good to take on training runs, spread in a sandwich. It's also good for longer races, for when you're tired of sweet things. Cashews contain high levels of magnesium, which is essential for healthy bone density and gives you a real boost during recovery.

CASHEW BUTTER

MAKES 1 X 225G (8OZ) JAR

200g (7oz) cashews, lightly roasted (see method)
1–2 tbsp neutral oil (optional)
a pinch of sea salt

1. Preheat the oven to 180°C/350°F/Gas 4.

2. Spread the nuts on a baking tray and roast for 8 minutes, then remove and allow to cool slightly.

3. Put the nuts into a high-powered food processor and blend until smooth. You can use a hand-held stick blender and a jug, but the result will be less smooth. You may need to add a little oil to help it along. Add a pinch of salt. It will keep for 2 weeks in a sealed container in the refrigerator.

Almonds are great for runners, as they are particularly high in vitamin E, an antioxidant that protects against toxins, and they deliver a punch of potassium, which encourages muscle recovery. I always use almonds with their skins on, just for a little extra fibre.

ALMOND BUTTER

MAKES 1 X 225G (8OZ) JAR

200g (7oz) skin-on almonds, lightly roasted (see method)
1–2 tbsp neutral oil (optional)
a pinch of sea salt

Follow the method for Cashew Butter, left.

Walnuts have a more bitter flavour than other nuts, so I add dates to bring a little sweetness. Walnuts are rich in omega 3 fatty acids, which help with inflammation and even prevent the breakdown of bone. Dates are a very fast-burning carbohydrate, which can give you a much-needed energy boost in a race.

WALNUT AND DATE BUTTER

MAKES 1 X 225G (8OZ) JAR

150g (5oz) shelled walnuts, lightly roasted (see method)
1–2 tbsp neutral oil (optional)
50g (2oz) pitted dates
a pinch of sea salt

Follow the method for Cashew Butter, left, but as the nuts begin to get smooth add the dates and a pinch of salt to the processor and blend further.

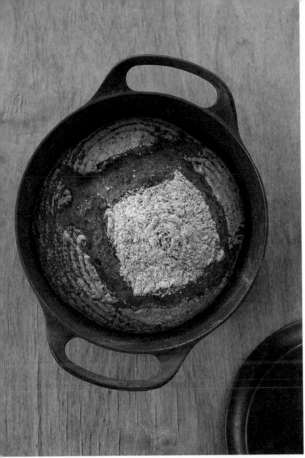

This is not really a recipe, just something that can be prepared quickly after an exhausting run. It is, perhaps, not something for everyday, but a welcome treat from time to time!

If you were to make this with standard white bread and store-bought peanut butter, the list of preservatives, sweeteners and additives would be almost endless, but here I count just five natural products! Enjoy.

NUT BUTTER AND BANANA ON TOAST

SERVES 4

8 slices of day-old Sourdough Bread (see p.185)
1 x quantity of Nut Butter (see p.199 – almond is my favourite)
4 bananas
honey, to taste
coarse sea salt, to taste

Toast the bread and liberally spread with the nut butter. Chop the bananas over the top, drizzle with honey and finish with a pinch of salt.

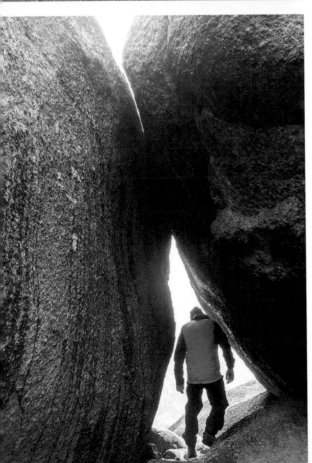

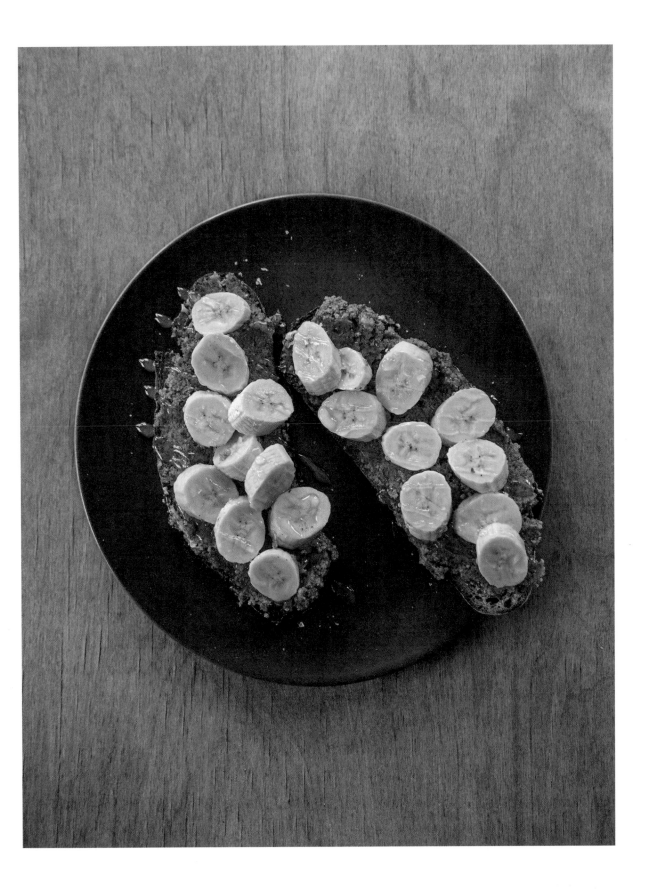

CHAPTER SIX

Drinks

———

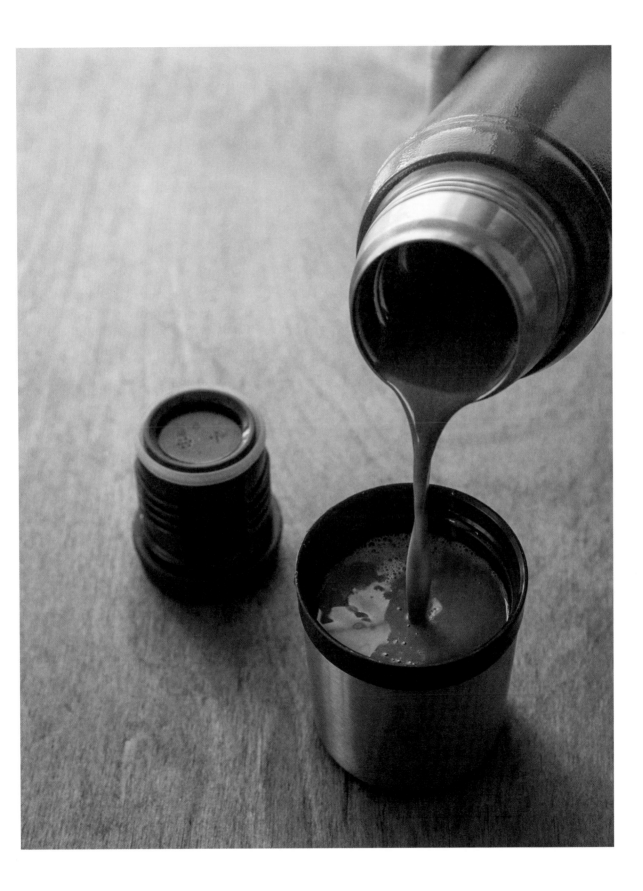

There certainly are health benefits to eating dark chocolate, but in this case the benefits are purely emotional! What better way to lift your spirits after a freezing cold winter run than a steaming cup of hot chocolate?

HOT CHOCOLATE

SERVES 4 (PICTURED ON P.203)

800ml (3¼ cups) milk (of your preferred choice)
100g (3¾oz) dark chocolate (minimum 70 per cent cocoa solids), broken up
3 tbsp maple syrup
1 tsp ground cinnamon (optional)

Combine the milk, chocolate and maple syrup in a saucepan and heat gently, stirring until the chocolate has completely melted and there are no lumps remaining. Bring it just to the boil, then it's ready to drink. You can add a spoonful of cinnamon, if you like that sort of thing.

I must admit I was extremely sceptical about turmeric latte when I first heard of it. I knew about the multitude of health benefits attributed to turmeric and it's a spice that I use often, but drinking it... no thank you! How wrong I was. Gently spiced and with a welcome bit of fire from the black pepper, it's a delicious way to start the day. You can use cow's milk, but the added coconut oil means it becomes too rich with full-fat or even semi-skimmed milk, so choose a low-fat skimmed milk for best results.

TURMERIC LATTE

SERVES 1

200ml (scant 1 cup) almond milk
½ tsp ground turmeric
½ tsp ground cinnamon
1 tsp honey
1 tsp coconut oil
2.5cm (1in) piece of fresh root ginger, coarsely chopped
a few grindings of black pepper (depending on how punchy you like it)

Combine all the ingredients in a saucepan and bring up to a gentle simmer. Simmer for 2 minutes, whisking from time to time until the ingredients have got to know one another. Strain the hot latte through a fine sieve into a waiting cup.

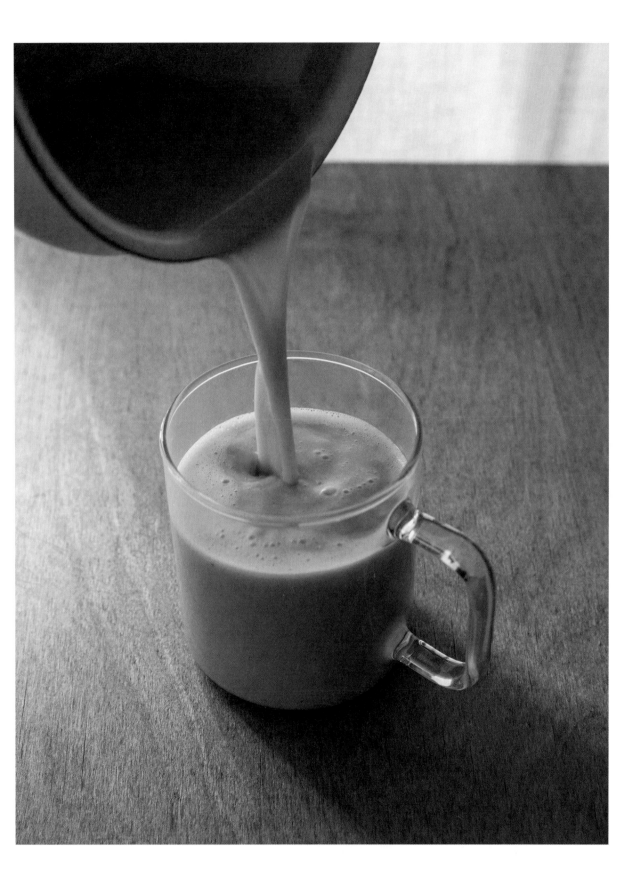

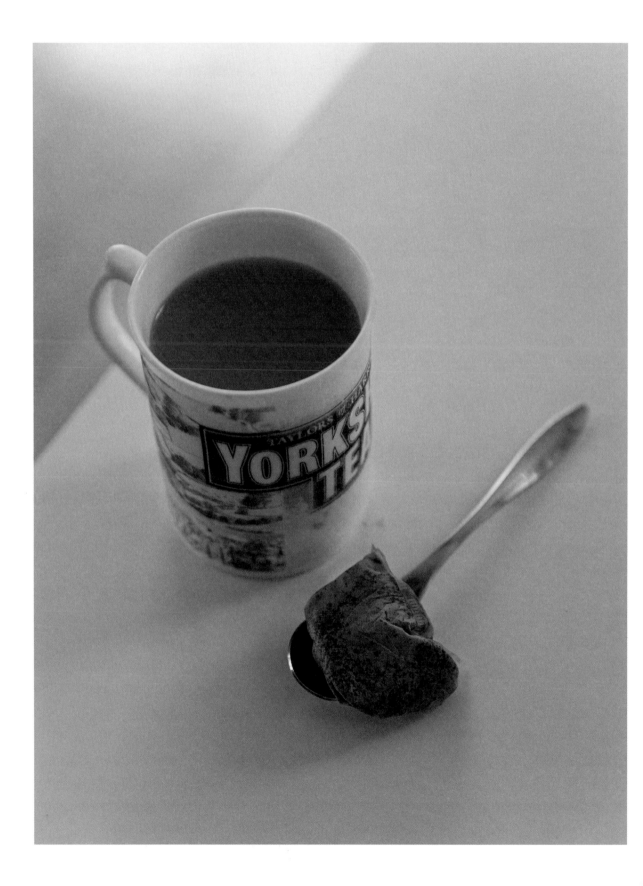

With a full-time job and a young family, one of the only ways I can manage to get in my base mileage every week is to run to work. It means an earlier start than I would like (5 a.m.), but it does allow for a steady 10km (6½-mile) run at the beginning of the day. It took a few weeks to fall into the routine of getting out of the door and running when I've barely opened my eyes, and in the dark Swedish winters my morning bed is especially hard to leave. However, after a couple of years of doing it, I couldn't imagine it any other way.

I've always been good at running on an empty stomach and I've never encountered any issues with doing a run before breakfast, but there's no way I'd get out of the house without a cup of tea beforehand. I don't know whether it has a placebo effect, or whether the caffeine and the calories from the splash of milk are in fact enough to sustain the journey, but I do know it makes me feel good and, at that time of the day, that's what matters.

STRONG BUILDER'S TEA

SERVES 1

1 English breakfast teabag (ideally Yorkshire, but others will suffice, at a push)

a drop of semi-skimmed milk

1. Put the tea bag in your favourite cup. Bring the kettle to the boil and pour the boiling water over the tea bag. Allow to mash for 2–3 minutes, then add a splash of milk and squeeze the teabag out with all the force you can muster, to make the tea as strong as possible.

2. Drink as soon as you can without burning yourself and get out the door before you can think of any excuses to get in the car or onto the bus.

Juices and Smoothies

Almost everyone of a certain age has a dusty juicer sitting at the back of a cupboard somewhere at home! We did too, until a few months ago. If you can get past the fact that cleaning a juicer after use is always a bit of a pain, I highly recommend getting into the habit of using them – it's a great way to get a lot of extra nutrients into your daily diet, as well as extra calories, which is important when training for long-distance running. If you don't have a juicer, these can also be made in a high-powered blender such as a Nutribullet; they will just be a little less smooth to drink (remember to add a little water when you blend).

These recipes are more of a guide than strict rules – experiment with your own juices and smoothies. Add blueberries to the Green Smoothie or melon to the Beetroot and Cucumber Juice to sweeten it up a bit, if you like. Most fruit and veg can be juiced. Although it's hard to give exact quantities, these recipes should yield two medium-sized servings. All juices are best consumed immediately, but will keep for one day in a sealed container in the refrigerator.

CUCUMBER, FENNEL, SPINACH AND APPLE JUICE

SERVES 2

½ cucumber, coarsely chopped
1 fennel bulb, coarsely chopped
2 apples, coarsely chopped
2 handfuls of spinach

Juice the cucumber, fennel and apple pieces, adding the spinach leaves halfway though the process and using a sturdy chunk of the fruit or veg to push it into the juicer.

BEETROOT AND CUCUMBER JUICE

SERVES 2

4 large beetroot, coarsely chopped
2 cucumbers, coarsely chopped

Just put everything through the juicer. This is the most hardcore juice in terms of flavour: it doesn't have as much natural sweetness as the other recipes and the earthiness of the beetroot can be an acquired taste.

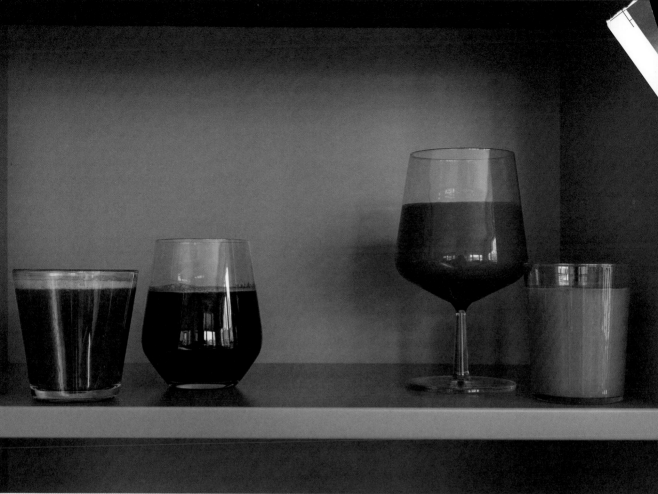

GREEN SMOOTHIE

SERVES 2

200ml (scant 1 cup) fresh apple juice, or extra as needed
a handful of kale
a handful of spinach
a handful of rocket (arugula)
50g (2oz) frozen mango chunks

Combine all the ingredients in a high-powered blender and blend to a smooth liquid. You may need to add a little more apple juice, if it's too thick.

CARROT, TURMERIC AND GINGER JUICE

SERVES 2

10 medium carrots, trimmed not peeled
50g (2oz) fresh root turmeric
50g (2oz) fresh root ginger

1. Juice half of the carrots, before putting the turmeric and ginger though the juicer. Finish with the final half of the carrots.

2. If you can't find fresh turmeric root, you could add 1 teaspoon ground turmeric at the end, or skip it – carrot and ginger is good too.

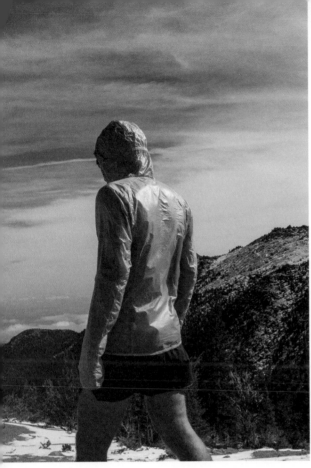

I often have this straight after a long training run. It's quick to make, delicious and full of the nutrients that your body is crying out for after training.

BANANA, ALMOND BUTTER AND CHIA SMOOTHIE

SERVES 1

1 ripe banana

1 tbsp chia seeds

1 tbsp almond butter (any nut butter will do, I just like almond best)

1 tsp honey

300ml (1¼ cups) milk (you can use almond or oat milk for a vegan version)

a pinch of sea salt

1. Put all the ingredients into a blender and blend until smooth.

2. Drink immediately. Oh, and rinse the glass straight away – it's a terrible pain to clean once dried!

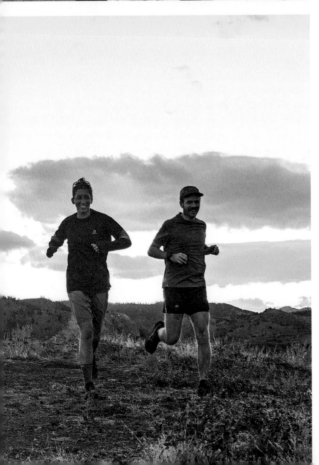

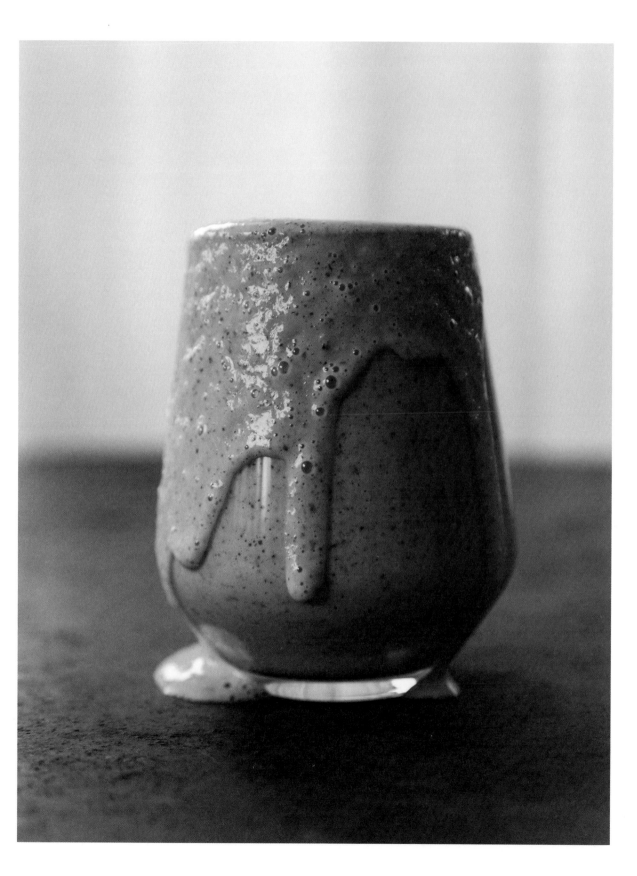

CHAPTER SEVEN

Snacks for Packs

———

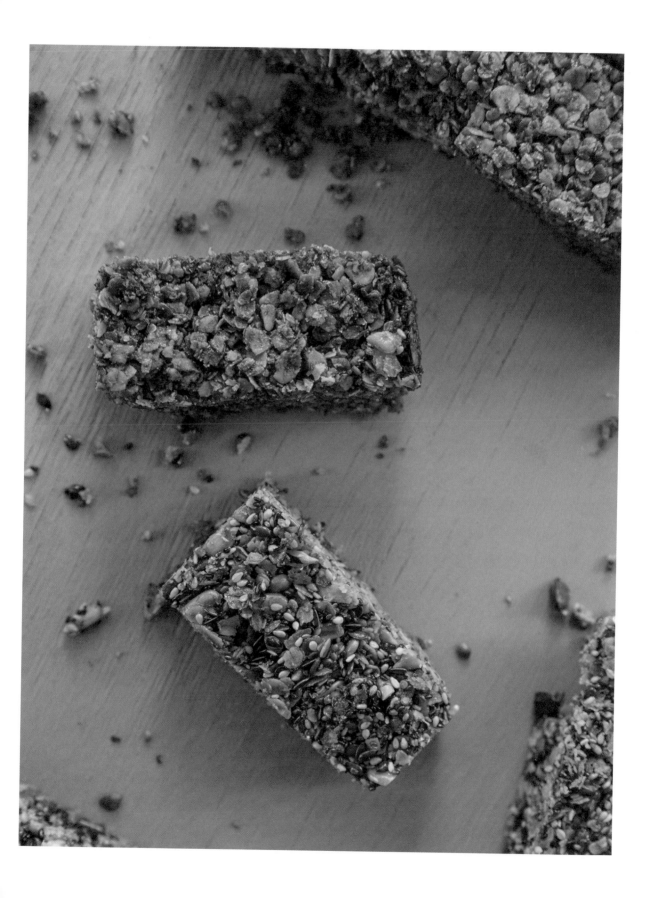

These bars make a nice change to those overly sweet cereal ones. The maple syrup binds everything together without making it too sweet and the chilli and thyme add an interesting touch (the chilli flakes give the bars a light warmth, but feel free to add more or less depending on your taste). Great to pack in the bag for a long day out on the trails, these are also always in my pack for longer races.

CHILLI AND THYME SEED BARS

MAKES 12 BARS

125g (4¼oz) rolled oats
125g (4¼oz) pumpkin seeds
50g (2oz) flax seeds (linseeds)
50g (2oz) chia seeds
50g (2oz) sesame seeds
1 tsp chopped thyme
½ tsp sea salt
½ tsp dried chilli flakes (or to taste)
100g (3¾oz) honey
100g (3¾oz) maple syrup
50ml (¼ cup) cold-pressed rapeseed oil

1. Preheat the oven to 180°C/350°F/Gas 4 and line a 20cm (8in) square deep baking tray with greaseproof paper.

2. Mix all the dry ingredients in a large bowl.

3. Combine the honey, maple syrup and rapeseed oil in a small saucepan and gently heat until the mixture becomes very runny and too hot to put your finger in. Pour the dry ingredients into the warm liquid and mix until well combined.

4. Evenly spread the mixture in the prepared baking tray, packing it down firmly. Bake for about 20 minutes until golden brown.

5. Remove the tray from the oven and cut the slab into bars while it is still warm, then allow to cool completely. The bars will keep for up to 2 weeks in a sealed container.

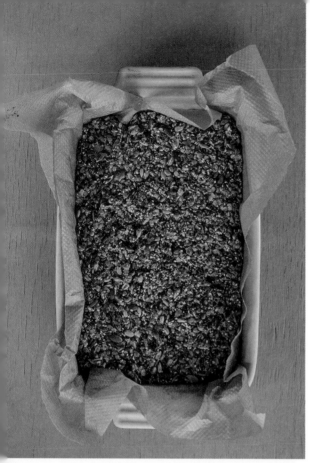

Before there were cereal bars there was the good old-fashioned flapjack! I love them and they're such a versatile and quick thing to make. Feel free to swap out the golden syrup for honey or maple syrup if you feel like it, or substitute the chocolate for nuts or raisins. Perfect before, during or after a long run, and quite nice when you're sitting on the sofa with a cup of tea just thinking about going out for a run!

CHOCOLATE FLAPJACK

MAKES 12 BARS

150g (5oz) golden syrup
200g (7oz) salted butter
100g (3¾oz) dark chocolate (minimum 70 per cent cocoa solids), broken up
350g (12oz) rolled oats
a pinch of sea salt

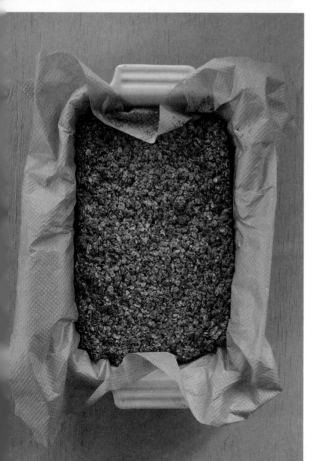

1. Preheat the oven to 180°C/350°F/Gas 4 and line a deep 20cm (8in) square baking tray with greaseproof paper.

2. In a heavy saucepan, heat the syrup, butter and chocolate over a low heat until the chocolate and butter have just melted. Add the oats and salt and mix well with a wooden spoon.

3. Pour the mixture into the prepared tray, spread it out evenly and firmly pat down. Bake for 15–18 minutes until lightly golden.

4. Allow to cool slightly, then cut into bars while still in the tray. Let it cool completely before eating. The bars will keep for up to a week stored in an airtight container.

Last year, I was asked if the kitchens at Rosendals Trädgård would provide some treats for the aid stations at the Ecotrail Stockholm race series. After some deliberation, our pastry chef Damien Boudet came up with this wonderful recipe. Baobab powder is available in most health food shops and a lot of supermarkets, and is high in fibre, vitamin C and many other micronutrients.

ECOTRAIL RAW SLICE

MAKES 12 BARS

125g (4¼oz) pitted dates
440g (scant 1lb) skin-on almonds
1 tbsp baobab powder
zest and juice of 1 lemon
120ml (½ cup) water
50g (2oz) flax seeds
50g (2oz) dried blueberries

1. Line a deep 20cm (8in) square baking tray with greaseproof paper or clingfilm.

2. Combine the dates, almonds, baobab powder, lemon zest and juice in a food processor and process until well blended, scraping down the side of the bowl from time to time. With the motor still running, slowly pour in the water through the feed tube until you have a smooth, thick, very sticky dough. Add the flax seeds and dried blueberries and pulse briefly just to mix them in.

3. Firmly press the mixture into the prepared baking tray, ensuring it is evenly spread out. Refrigerate overnight or for at least 4–5 hours, then slice into bars. The bars will keep well for up to a week, stored in an airtight container in the refrigerator.

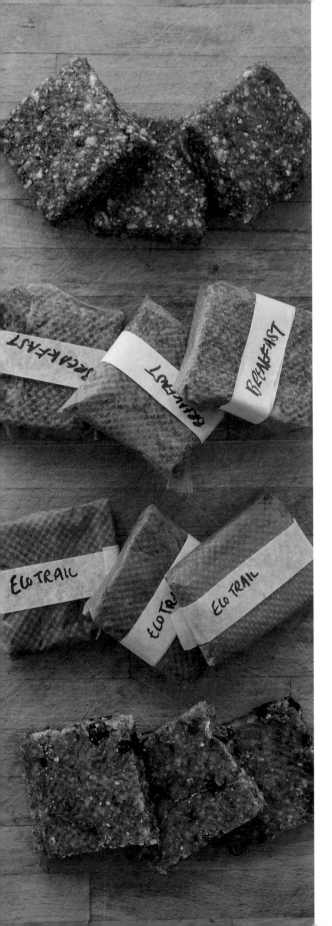

This recipe is a slight reworking from the fantastic *River Cottage Light and Easy*; a book I highly recommend. They make a great quick breakfast, but are also very useful to take out on a run. They do tend to get a bit soft, so are best eaten early in the run rather than later.

RAW BREAKFAST SLICE

MAKES 10 BARS

100g (3¾oz) rye or oat flakes
75g (2½oz) skin-on almonds
170g (6oz) dried apricots
200g (7oz) pitted dates
50g (2oz) raisins
2 dried figs, stems removed
zest and juice of 1 orange

1. Line a 20cm (8in) square deep baking tray with greaseproof paper or clingfilm.

2. Put all the ingredients except the orange juice into a food processor and pulse until well chopped and combined, stopping from time to time to scrape down the sides. Slowly add the orange juice and pulse until you get a thick, chunky paste.

3. Firmly press the mixture into the prepared baking tray, ensuring it is evenly spread out. Refrigerate overnight or for at least 4–5 hours until firm, then slice into bars. The bars keep well for up to 2 weeks, stored in a airtight container in the refrigerator.

This is something I carry with me on all long runs, and especially longer races, when you can take it a bit easy from time to time (I don't recommend trying to run quickly while munching on a mouthful of nuts and berries). I find the crunch and saltiness is a welcome change from the sweet things that I often eat when I'm out for a long day.

TRAIL MIX

MAKES ENOUGH FOR A COUPLE OF LONG RUNS

100g (3¾oz) almonds
100g (3¾oz) walnuts
100g (3¾oz) cashews
a drizzle of olive oil
a pinch of sea salt
2 tbsp maple syrup (optional)
50g (2oz) dried cranberries
50g (2oz) dried blueberries
30g (1⅕oz) coconut flakes

1. Preheat the oven to 180°C/350°F/Gas 4.

2. Put the nuts into a bowl and drizzle with a little olive oil and a big pinch of sea salt, stirring to coat. You can also add maple syrup at this point, if you are feeling a bit luxurious. Spread the nuts over a baking tray and toast in the oven until lightly golden, about 8 minutes.

3. Allow the nuts to cool completely, then mix with the berries and coconut flakes.

4. The mixture will keep well for at least 2 weeks in a sealed jar or a zip-lock bag.

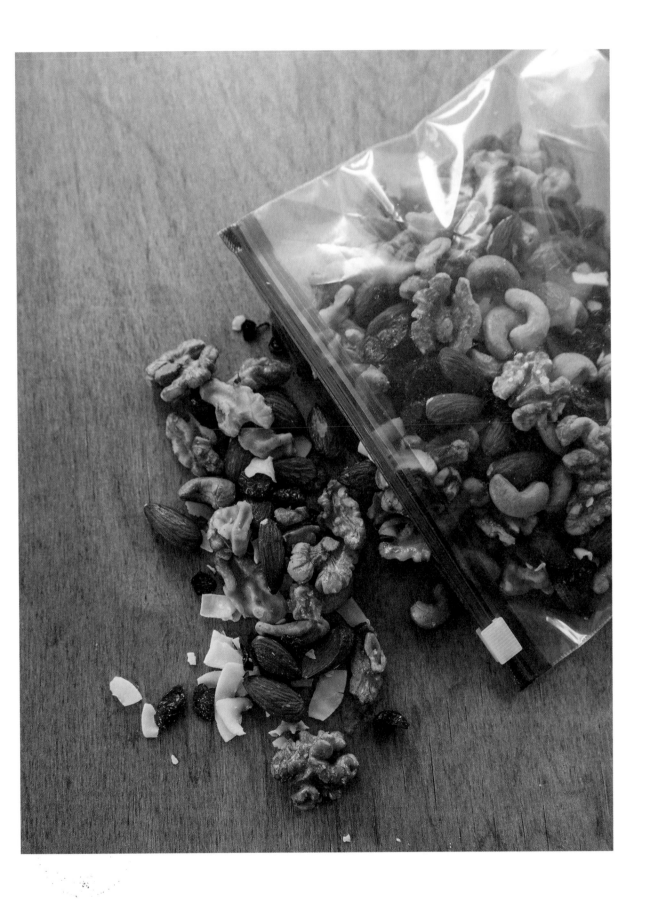

Index to Recipes

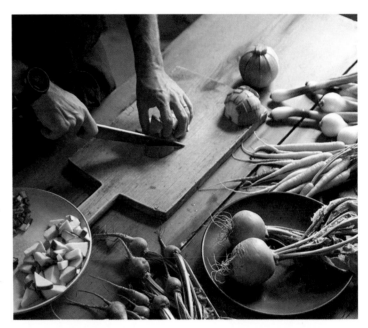

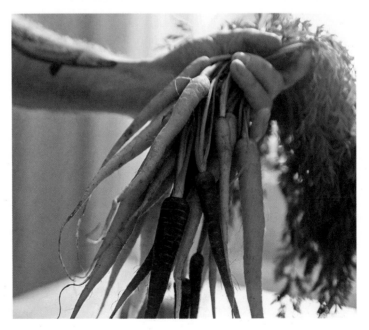

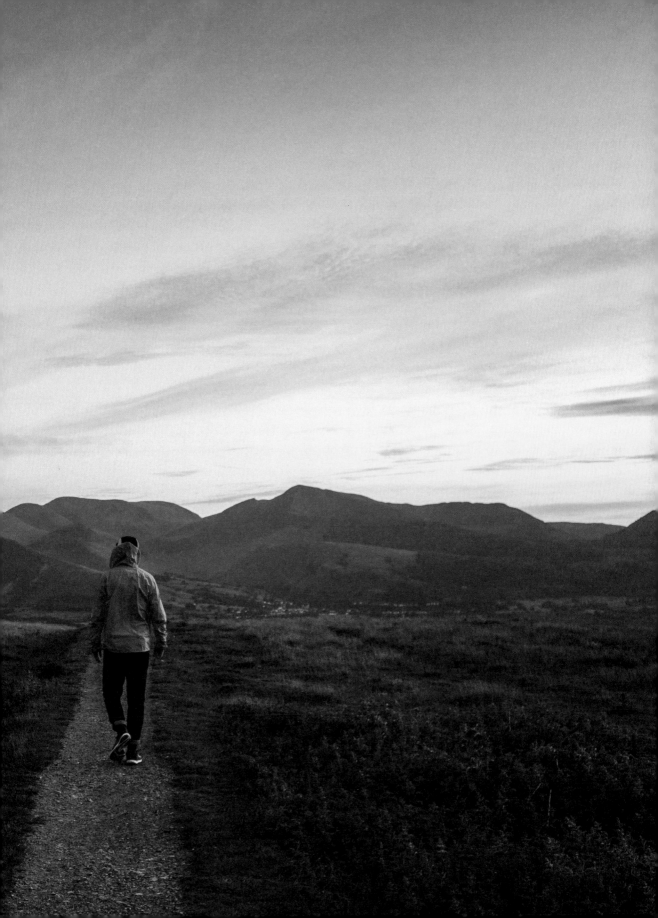

Thank You

To the many chefs and cooks who have influenced and helped shape me
as a cook over the years. There are too many of you to mention and every one
of you is important

The staff at Rosendals Trädgård for making it a pleasure to go to work every day

Charlotte and Patrik at Gawell Förlag for taking a chance on me

Emily, guiding me through my first steps as a writer

Kai for his Jedi design skills

All the wonderful suppliers who helped make this possible, Anna & David
at Sorunda Grönsakshallen, Maria & Lena at Ekofisk & Susanne at Smorgasbord,
without your help it would never have been possible

Ciele Athletics for providing me with the best hats in the business

Cahir for challenging me to that first half marathon, Chris for being open to
some of the biggest challenges, Petter for getting me out the door when I'm not
feeling like it. Everyone at Team Nordic Trail for helping me become a better
runner and the countless others in the running community whom
I've shared miles with over the years

Mum and dad for being there even though I am often far away

Walter and Mimmi for giving me perspective about what's really important in life

For Christin, I can't thank you enough, I can't imagine life without you by my side

About the Author

Billy White is a British chef based in Sweden, who has a background in fine dining,
including St. John in London, Fäviken and Restaurant Mathias Dahlgren.
He is now head chef at Rosendals Trädgård, Stockholm